Health Care

FOR BEGINNERS

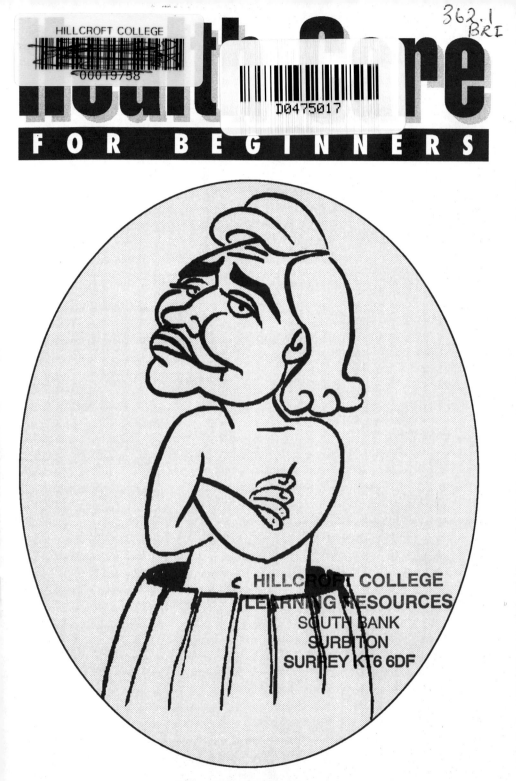

By David Brizer
Illustrated by Ricardo Castaneda

WRITERS AND READERS PUBLISHING, INC.

P.O. Box 461, Village Station
New York, NY 10014

Writers and Readers Limited
9 Cynthia Street
London N1 9JF
England

•

A Writers and Readers Documentary Comic Book
Copyright © 1994

ISBN # 0-86316-170-7 Trade
1 2 3 4 5 6 7 8 9 0

Manufactured in the United States of America

Beginners Documentary Comic Books are published by Writers and Readers
Publishing, Inc. Its trademark, consisting of the words "For Beginners, Writers and
Readers Documentary Comic Books" and the Writers and Readers logo, is registered
in the U. S. Patent and Trademark Office and in other countries.

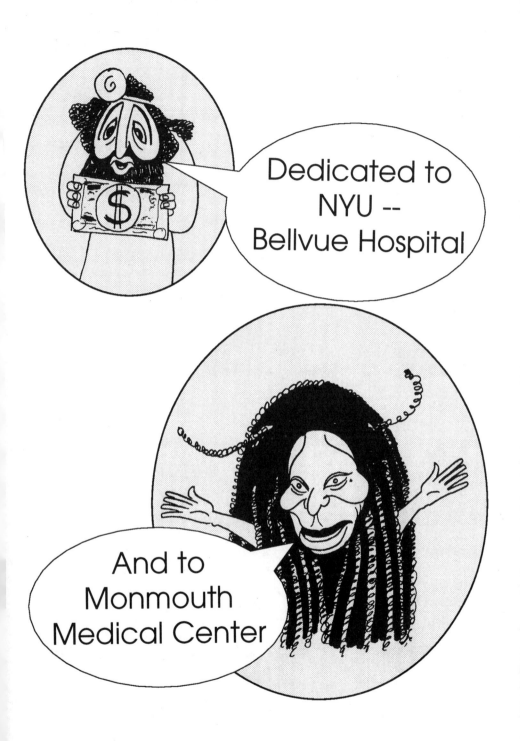

CONTENTS

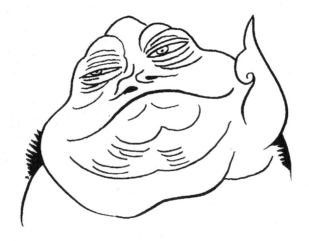

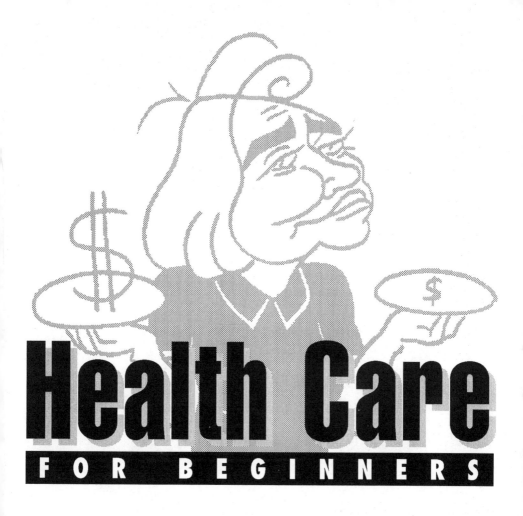

Health Care

FOR BEGINNERS

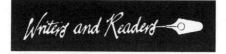

Writers and Readers

PRIMUM NON NOCERE*

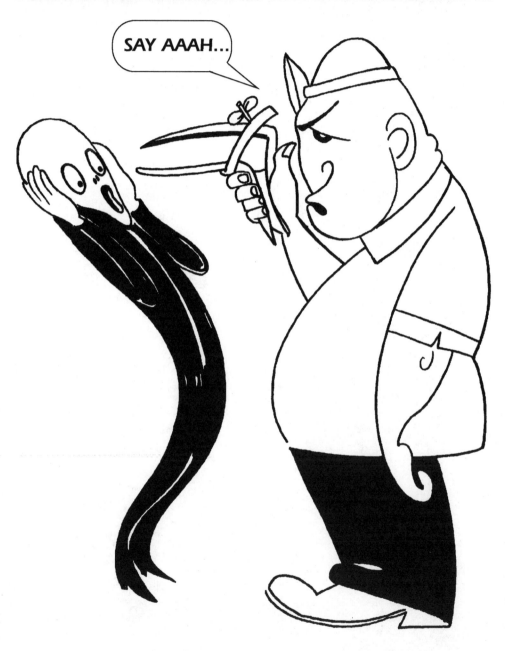

("First, do no harm.")

What would you do if **you** needed an autologous bone marrow transplant?

Or TPA (Tissue Plasminogen Activator)—at a mere $2200 a dose?

Or ceredase treatments for Gaucher's disease, at an approximate cost of $200,000 per year?

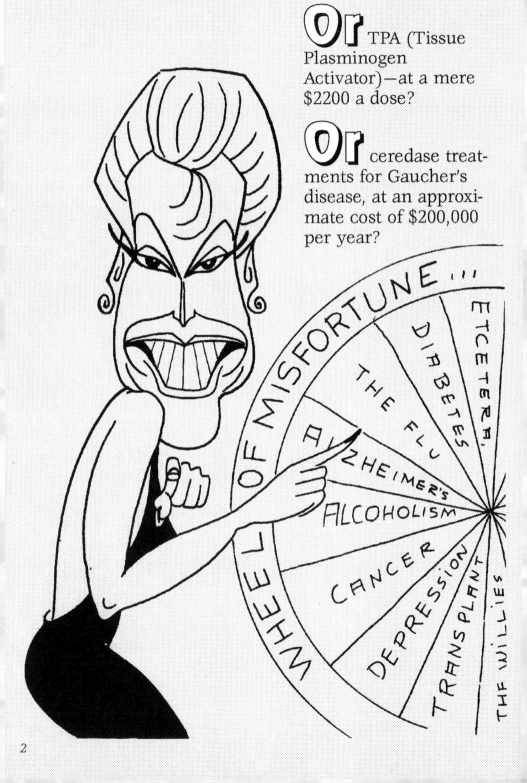

Or what if you needed extended treatment for depression or alcoholism? Could you afford it?

Could your wallet survive any of these?

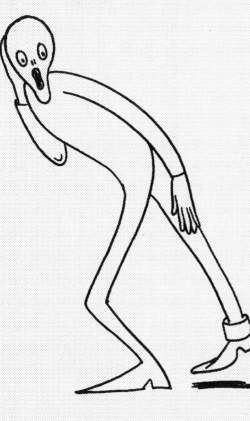

For most of us, who aren't millionaires and don't have superb medical insurance, the answer is a loud and resounding

BILL $

NO.

Fact is, many people don't know which conditions are covered by their health insurance.

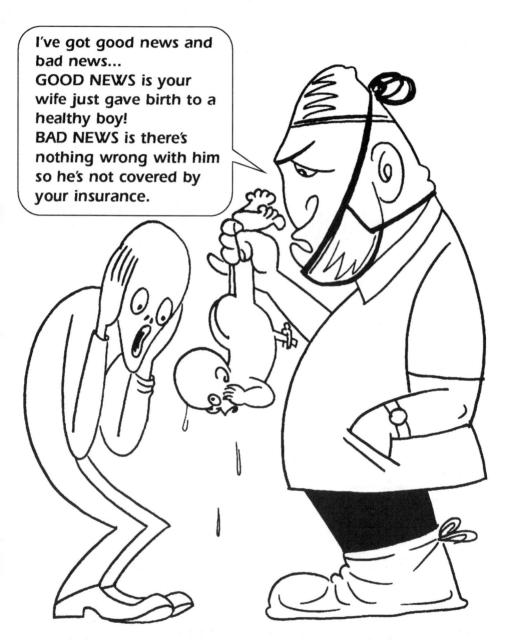

Even more don't know which conditions are *excluded* from coverage by their policies...and this often comes as a rude awakening, at the worst possible time—when illness strikes.

If you *have* medical insurance, that is.

Some thirty-seven million people in this country do not.

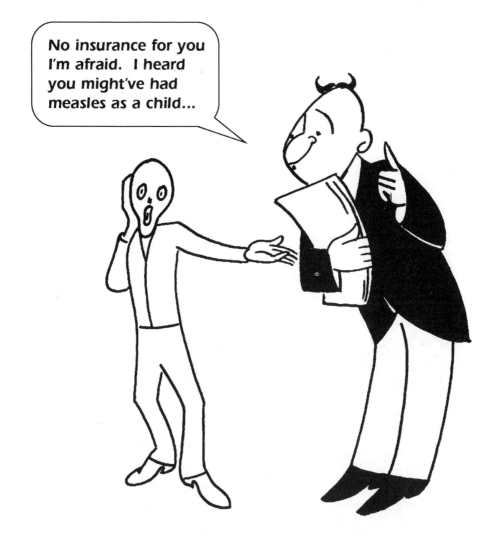

Two million are considered "uninsurable" because of pre-existing disorders.

The number of uninsured Americans increased by about 7 million from 1980 to 1989.

Those who have low paying jobs in small companies often have no medical insurance. Other companies may provide health benefits to workers but not to their families. Students past their teens are also a highly uninsured group.

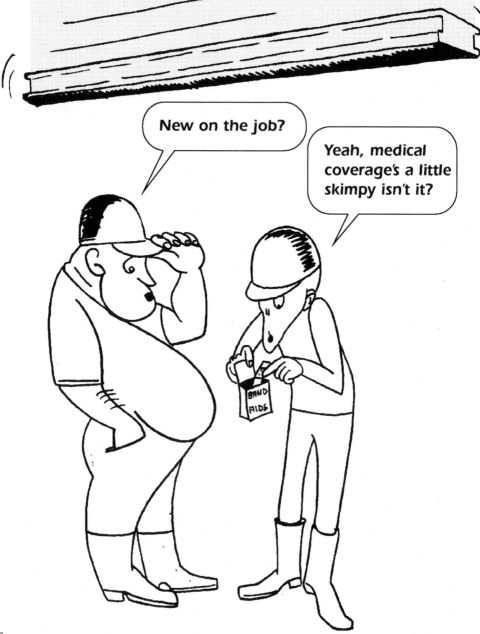

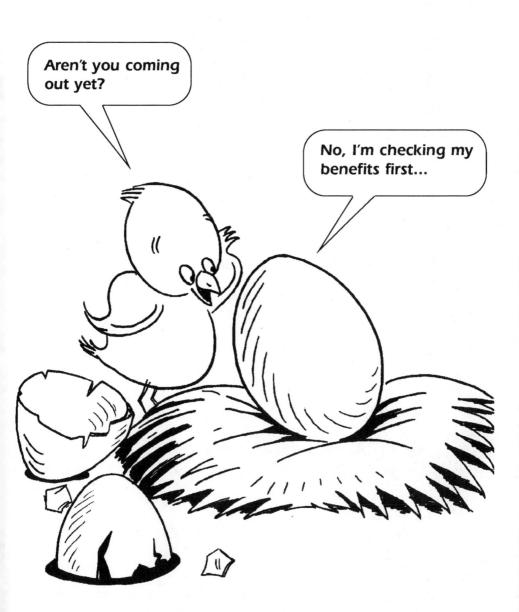

Eighteen percent of the
children in this country have no medical insurance.

Did you know that the U.S., along with South Africa, are unique among industrialized nations in not guaranteeing health care access for all their citizens?

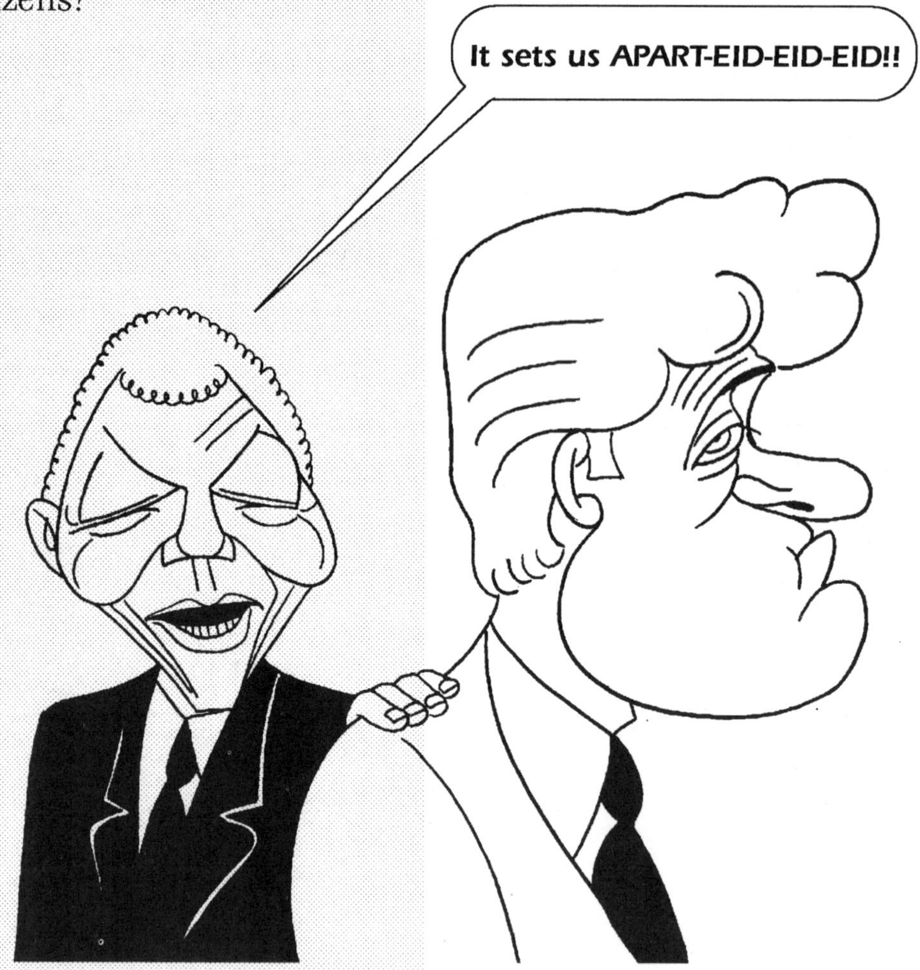

Yet the U.S. has among the highest physician-to-patient ratios of all countries.

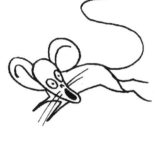

If the answers to any of these questions come as a surprise, then this book is for you. Read on...and may you always remain healthy....

HEALTH CARE FOR BEGINNERS:
A Postmodern Morality Play

Starring
(in order of appearance):

★ Mrs. Hillary Rodham Clinton

★ Dr. Donald Dollerz

★ Dr. George Goodheart

★ Mr. Poindexter Prufrock, insurance company executive

★ Mr. Noah Nostrum, drug manufacturer

★ Ms. Doris Brown, citizen and mother of three

...and a cast of millions.

Donald Dollerz, M.D.

Born with a cellular phone glued to his ear. Couldn't decide between orthopedics or plastics—so he does both. Favorite reading: his bank book. Goal in life: to finance world's first 18-hole golf course/orthopedic institute.

Hillary Rodham Clinton

Progressive, pro-egalitarian, pro-feminist; a humanitarian attorney(!); brilliant but real—the current First Lady—but most definitely not a Barbara or Nancy clone.

George Goodheart, M.D.

Always ribbed by his schoolmates for his credo ("*I want to help as many people as I can.*") as well as for his choice of specialty (family practice). A gentleman and a scholar. Doesn't openly admit it, but has been known to *actually make* house calls.

Poindexter Prufrock
(CEO, SMEGMA Insurance Co.)

This blue-blooded "Good Old Boy" is the genuine article, hailing from a long line of Republicans who live and die by the "trickle down" theory (for every million he makes, he'll let a buck or two "trickle on down").
Articulate, glib, patronizing-still boasts about the time he sold insurance to his neighbor's dog.

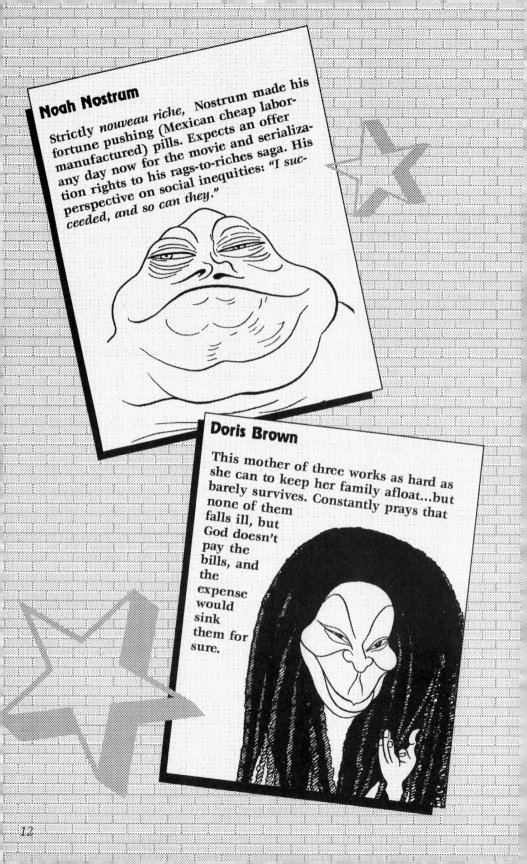

Noah Nostrum

Strictly *nouveau riche*, Nostrum made his fortune pushing (Mexican cheap labor-manufactured) pills. Expects an offer any day now for the movie and serialization rights to his rags-to-riches saga. His perspective on social inequities: *"I succeeded, and so can they."*

Doris Brown

This mother of three works as hard as she can to keep her family afloat...but barely survives. Constantly prays that none of them falls ill, but God doesn't pay the bills, and the expense would sink them for sure.

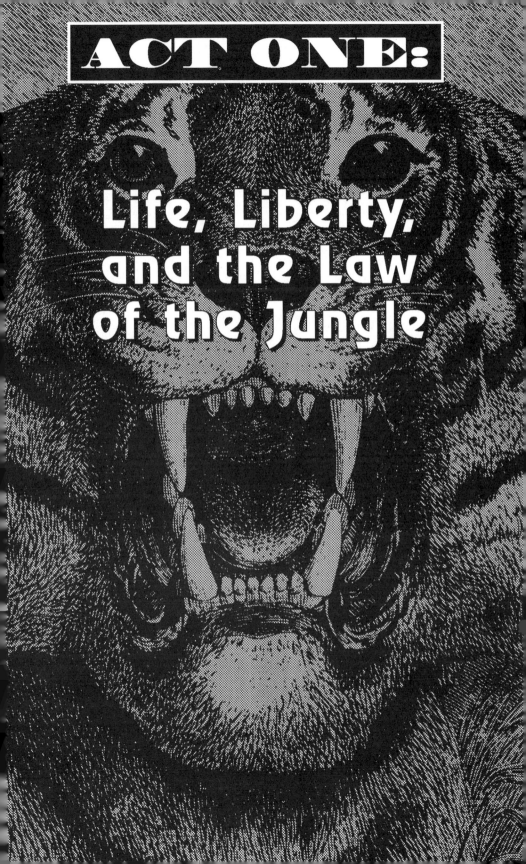

ACT ONE:

Life, Liberty, and the Law of the Jungle

"So you insist on universal education, but not universal health care."

"Imagine proposing that schools should only be for those who can pay for it."

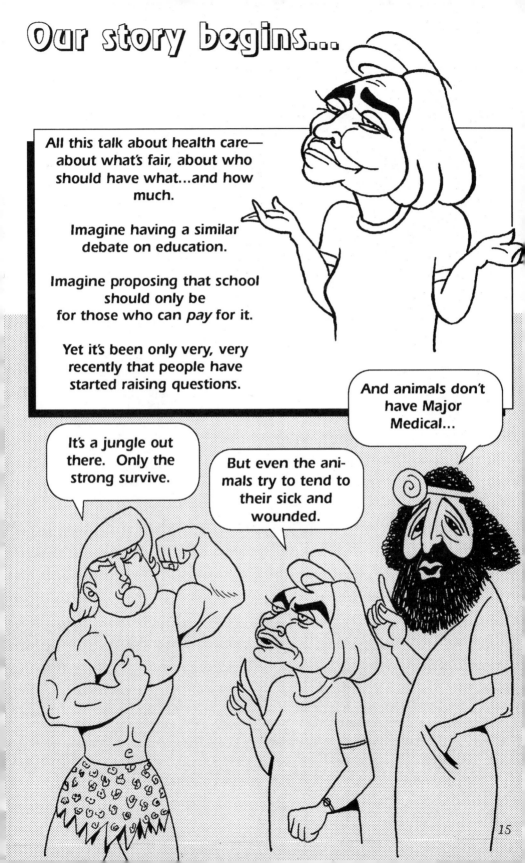

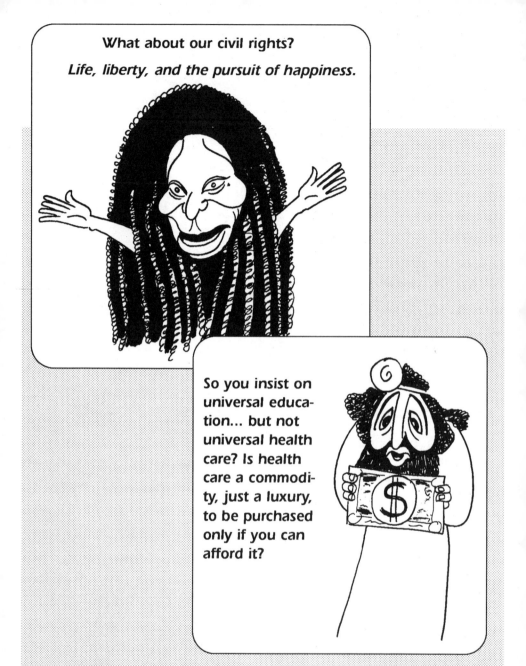

Health care *is* different from other commodities. You never know when you'll need it; it's usually not optional; and most of the time consumers have very little or no say in the services they actually receive...and very little awareness of the ultimate price of the services they buy.

What can we do?

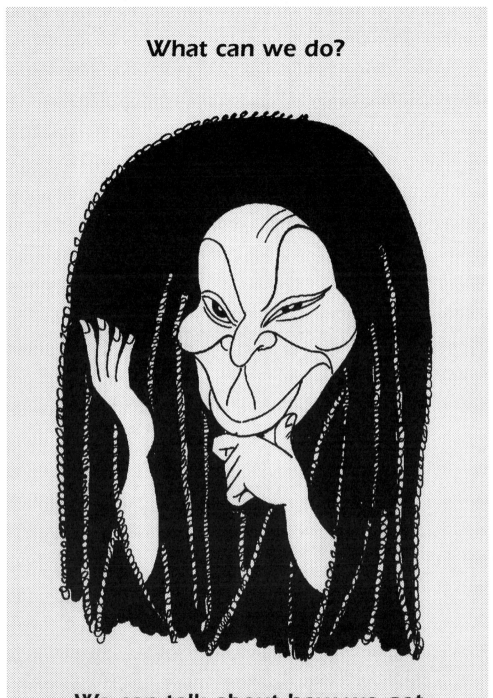

We can talk about how we got
here, about which systems
seem to work and which don't.

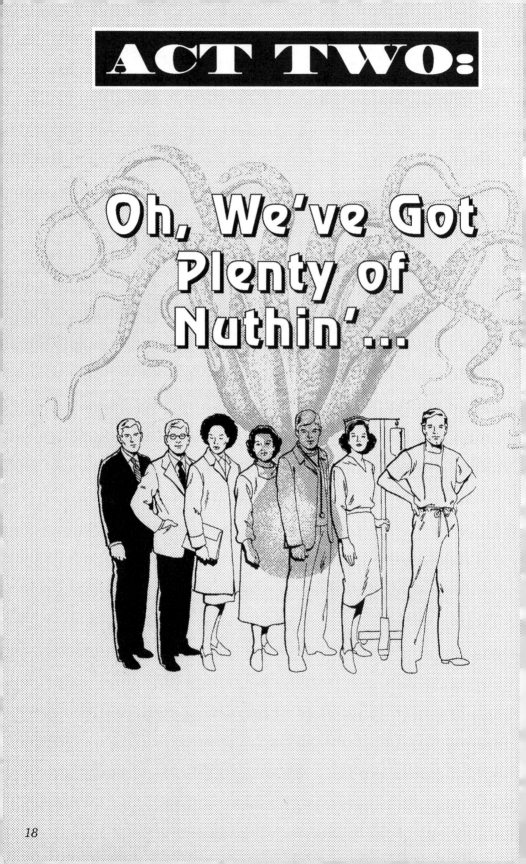

ACT TWO:

Oh, We've Got Plenty of Nuthin'...

"Those between the ages of 20 and 30 and those over 65 have the most illnesses and the greatest need for health care."

"Chronic illness presents the greatest cost to society: 86% of those over the age of 65 have one or more chronic illnesses."

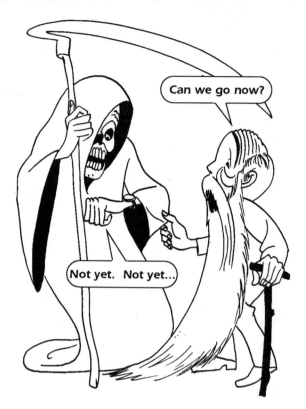

The life span of the average American has increased dramatically in this century.

Now that people live longer, *chronic* illnesses are more prevalent.

Chronic illness presents the greatest cost to society: 86% of those over the age of 65 have one or more chronic illnesses.

The three most frequent illnesses of old age are arthritis, hypertension, and heart disease. Young people are more likely to develop acute conditions such as colds, influenza, and injuries.

Those between the ages of 20 and 30 and those over 65 have the most illnesses and the greatest need for health care.

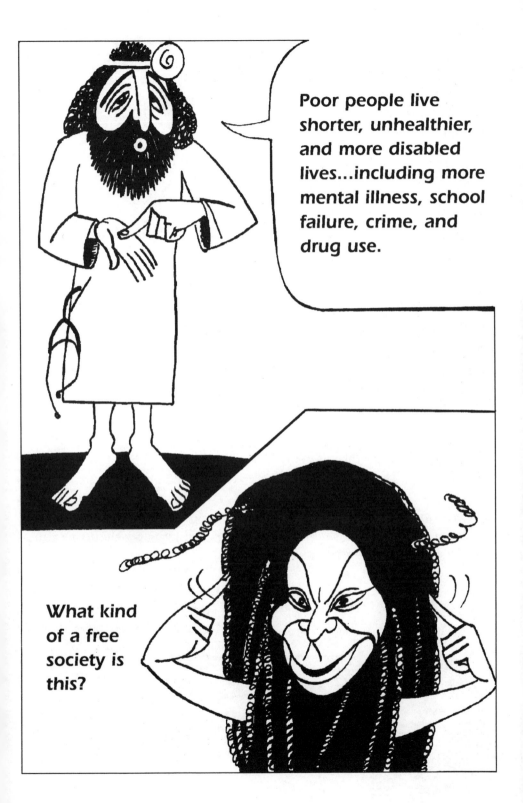

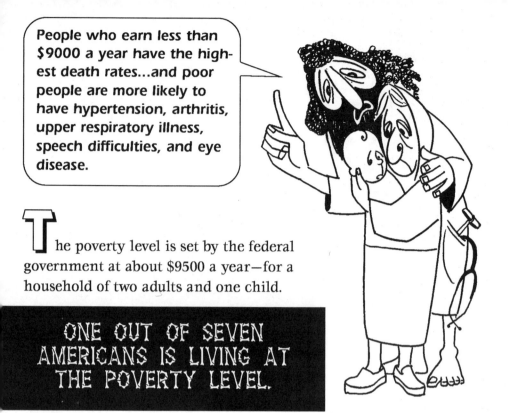

People who earn less than $9000 a year have the highest death rates...and poor people are more likely to have hypertension, arthritis, upper respiratory illness, speech difficulties, and eye disease.

The poverty level is set by the federal government at about $9500 a year—for a household of two adults and one child.

ONE OUT OF SEVEN AMERICANS IS LIVING AT THE POVERTY LEVEL.

Race affects the rate of visits to health care providers. African Americans make proportionally fewer visits to doctors than whites.

African Americans had a death rate almost 50% (42.5%, according to the Department of Health and Human Services) greater than the population average between 1979-81.

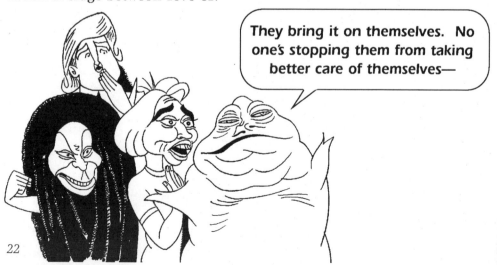

They bring it on themselves. No one's stopping them from taking better care of themselves—

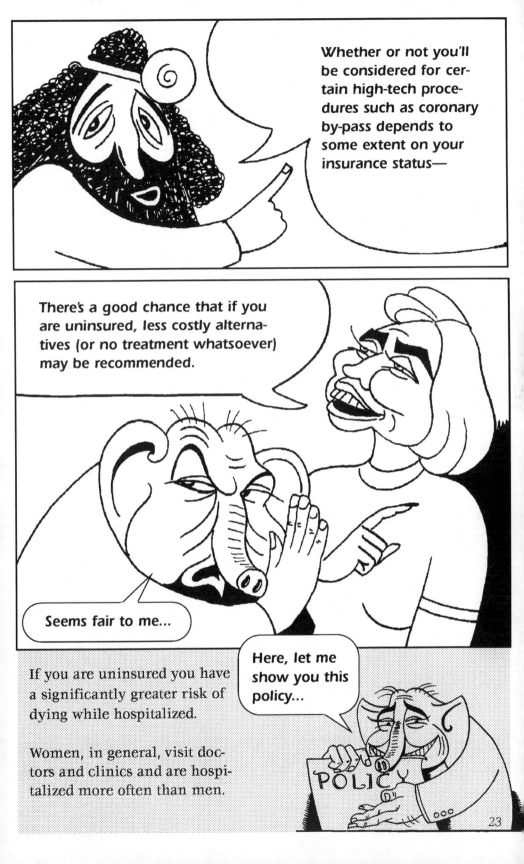

Whether or not you'll be considered for certain high-tech procedures such as coronary by-pass depends to some extent on your insurance status—

There's a good chance that if you are uninsured, less costly alternatives (or no treatment whatsoever) may be recommended.

Seems fair to me...

If you are uninsured you have a significantly greater risk of dying while hospitalized.

Women, in general, visit doctors and clinics and are hospitalized more often than men.

Here, let me show you this policy...

POLICY

23

And then there's pollution. Slowly but surely, we're poisoning ourselves to death. One estimate is that the *environment* contributes to about one-quarter of today's medical problems.

Infant mortality in the U.S. compares poorly with that of other countries, with the U.S. ranked in 21st place.

The mortality rate for black infants is twice as high as for white infants. Low infant mortality is associated with good prenatal care; while approximately 80% of white mothers receive prenatal care, only 65% of black mothers do.

Statistics, shmapistics...Anyone for golf?

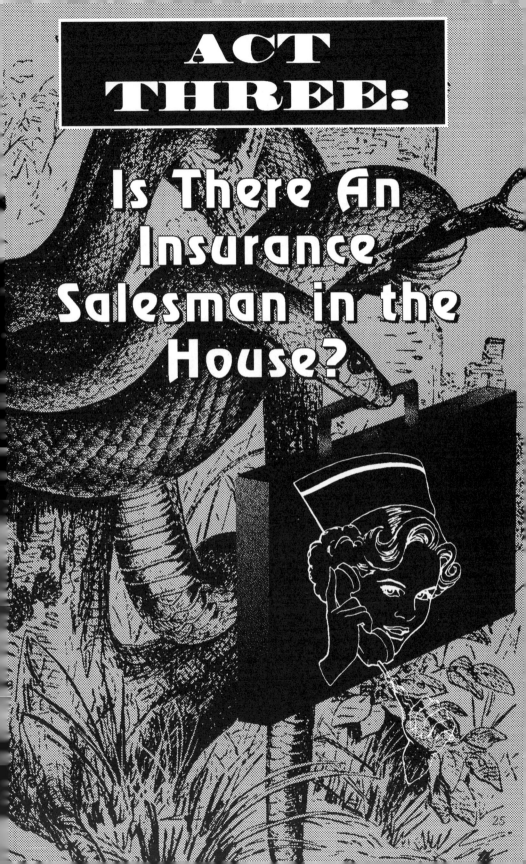

ACT THREE:

Is There An Insurance Salesman in the House?

"Other countries spend
less and do better."

"In Canada, Great
Britain, France, and
Germany the size of the
health care bite out of
the GNP remains the
same from year to year."

So the whole thing's a big rotten mess. How did things *get* so screwed up?

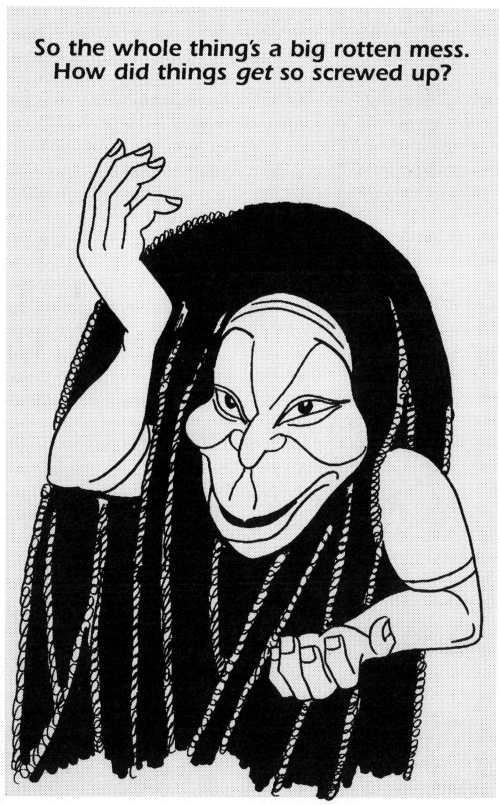

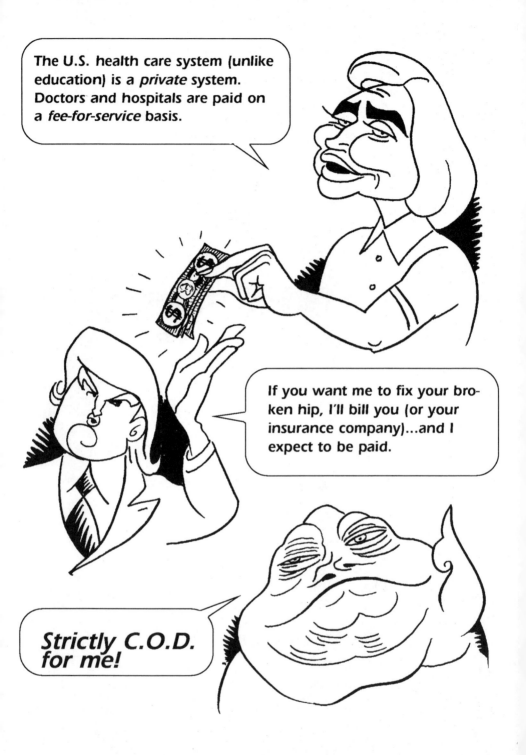

There are about 600,000 practicing physicians in the U.S. today, along with 130,000 dentists and 1.5 million nurses. One-third of the physicians are in primary care (general practitioners, family practice, internists, and pediatricians).

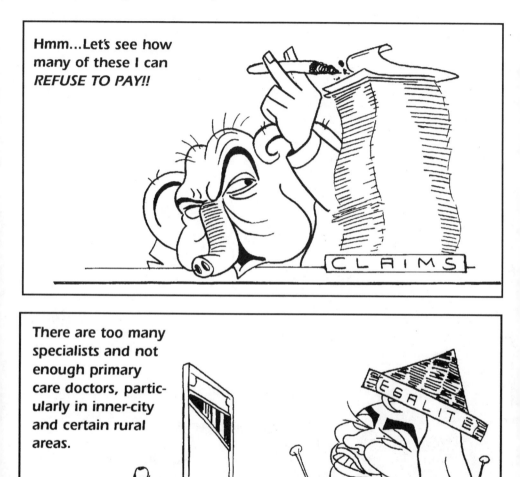

Tell me about it. And tell me this: Is anyone in charge? Is there anyone looking over the shoulders of this army of docs?

Certain *regulatory agencies* oversee hospital standards and service delivery. Chief among these is JCAHO (Joint Commission on Accreditation of Hospitals), which inspects hospitals every two years for compliance with its own standards of quality.

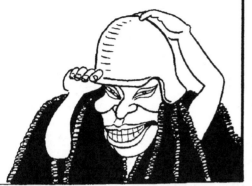

Without JCAHO accreditation, federal reimbursement to hospitals from Medicare and Medicaid is withheld—

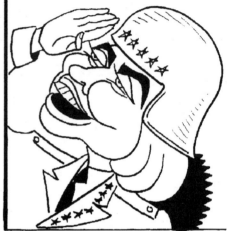

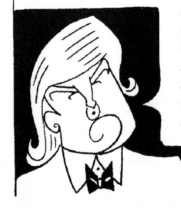

Federal reimbursement he cares about...

—so JCAHO has a great deal to say about how hospitals are run. Hospitals must also operate within standards set by city and state governmental agencies.

The Federal Health Care Financing Administration (HCFA) is responsible for federally funded health care financing (principally Medicare and Medicaid).

Patients pay for services directly out of pocket or more commonly through *third-party payers*— insurance companies, that is.(The first two parties are the patient and the doctor.)

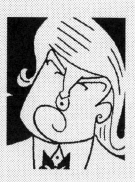

First party, second party, third party... all these *parties*... how come *I* never get invited?

Most of the private insurance coverage in America is paid for by employers (2/3 of American workers' health coverage is through their employer)...

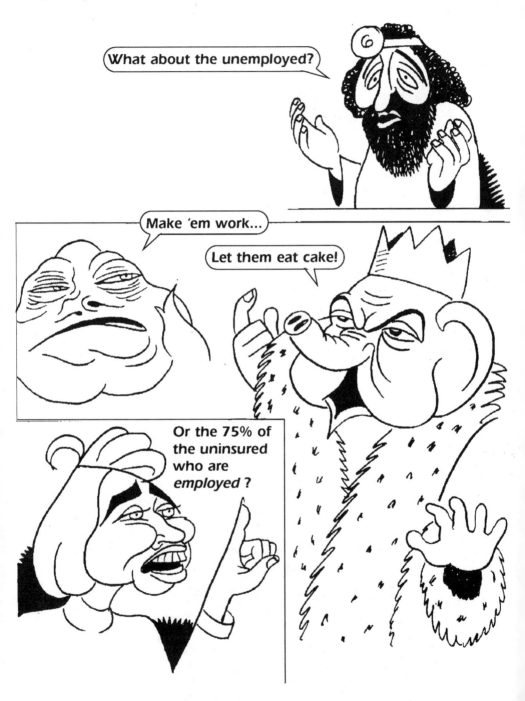

The traditional arrangement has been for third-party payers to provide reimbursement to doctors, hospitals, and/or patients *retrospectively:* the doctor, or the dentist, or the hospital submits the bill for services (*fee for service*) to the insurance company and is paid later on.

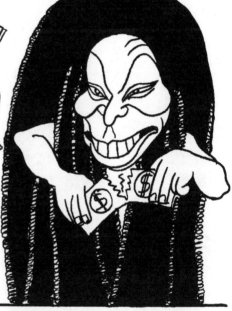

Most policies only cover *part* of the bill; most policies have *deductibles,* which is the amount the patient must pay before the insurance coverage kicks in to cover part or all the rest of the expense (= *cost sharing*).

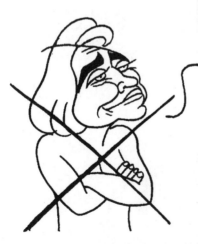

One effect of cost sharing is that the poor—particularly poor children—get even less access to needed health care. Some services, such as treatment for mental health or dental care, may not be covered at all.

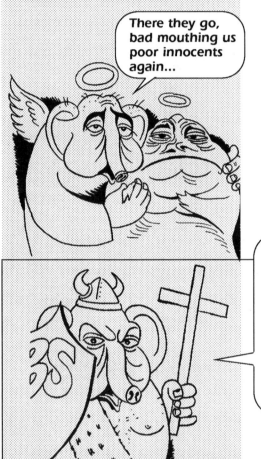

aybe this helps explain why Americans see doctors less often than people in other countries, such as France or Germany, where national health systems help pay for most medical care.

There they go, bad mouthing us poor innocents again...

Speaking of third-party payers... Who *are* the major third-party payer players?

The Blue Cross (*Blue Cross/Blue Shield*) Association is a group of over 80 independent insurance plans nationwide. Blue Cross pays for hospital stays; Blue Shield pays for hospital-related doctors' bills. When Blue Cross was the nation's major health insurer, Blue Cross fees could be based on *community rating* ...

Excuse Me !

With community rating, health care costs of entire communities were averaged, so that those with major health (= expensive) health care needs could be covered as well as those with little or no health expenses.

By the early 1950s, private commercial insurers, covering lower-risk individuals at reduced fees, had come to dominate the industry.

By the end of the 1980s, commercial insurers like Prudential, Aetna, Metropolitan, and Cigna (and about 1500 others) handled 40% of the market; unlike Blue Cross, these companies are out to make a profit.

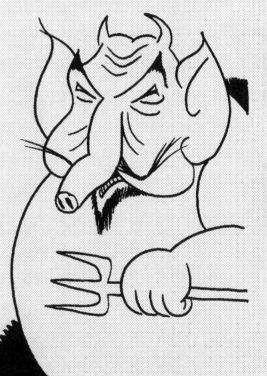

owadays, about a third of the nation's health insurance is handled by companies that *self-insure* (work out health insurance arrangements privately or use established insurance companies as administrators).

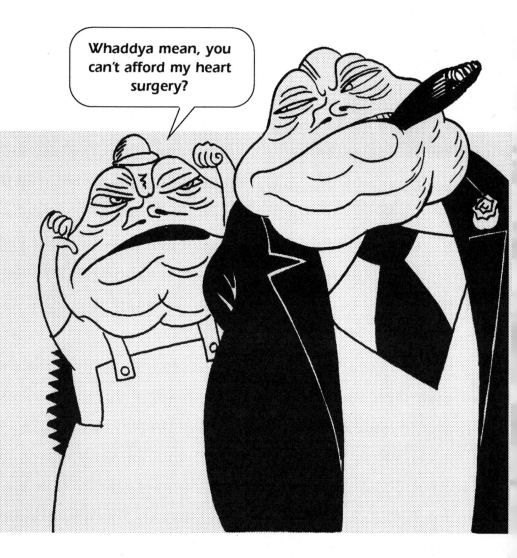

Medicare (Title 18.)

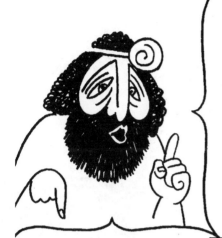

Created by the Federal Social Security Act of 1965, Medicare provides both hospital and medical insurance for those over 65 years of age and for those with certain disabilities (such as blindness or kidney disease). Part A of Medicare pays for inpatient hospital care, home health services, dialysis, and nursing home care after hospitalization.

Medicare Part A originates from Social Security contributions we pay in our income tax.

Part B is optional medical insurance that can be purchased to cover services like doctors' fees, medical supplies, home health care, outpatient hospital care, and therapy services.

Benefits and eligibility standards for Medicare are uniform throughout the United States. Currently, more than 33 million people are covered by Medicare.

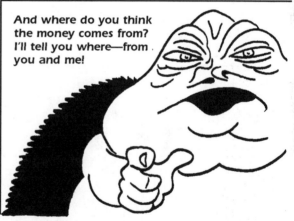

And where do you think the money comes from? I'll tell you where—from you and me!

Outpatient prescriptions, nursing home care, and hearing aids are not covered under Medicare.

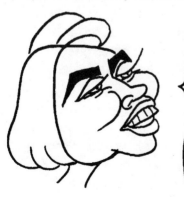

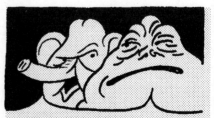

Thank heaven for small favors...

Medicaid (Title 19.)

Medicaid, an assistance program for needy and low-income people—

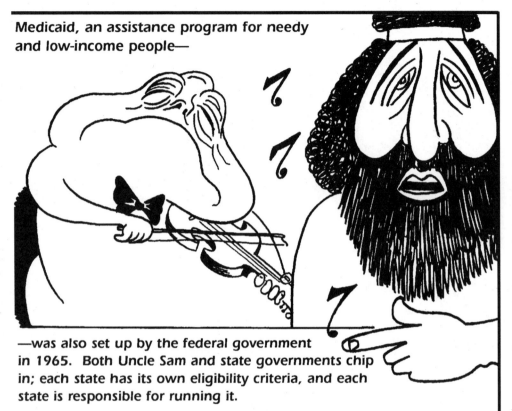

—was also set up by the federal government in 1965. Both Uncle Sam and state governments chip in; each state has its own eligibility criteria, and each state is responsible for running it.

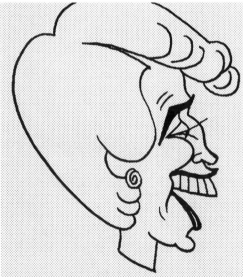

About 24 million people are currently covered by Medicaid.

In order to qualify for Medicaid, people must often completely use up their personal funds. Increasingly tight eligibility requirements (such as needing to qualify for welfare) have left more and more low- and no-income people without coverage.

Medicaid is no bargain. In order to qualify, not only do you have to be poor—

—in some states, what is considered 'poor' is far below the federal poverty standard—

—but you may also have to meet other specific state standards, such as being a single parent.

Might as well insist that you have zebra stripes or two heads.

I LIKE IT, I LIKE IT...

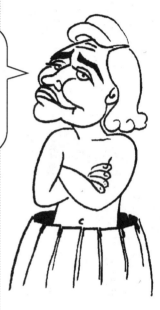

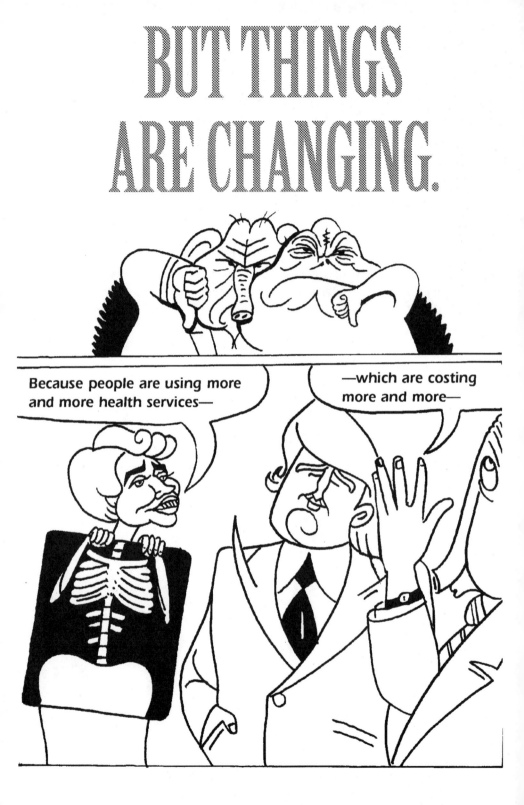

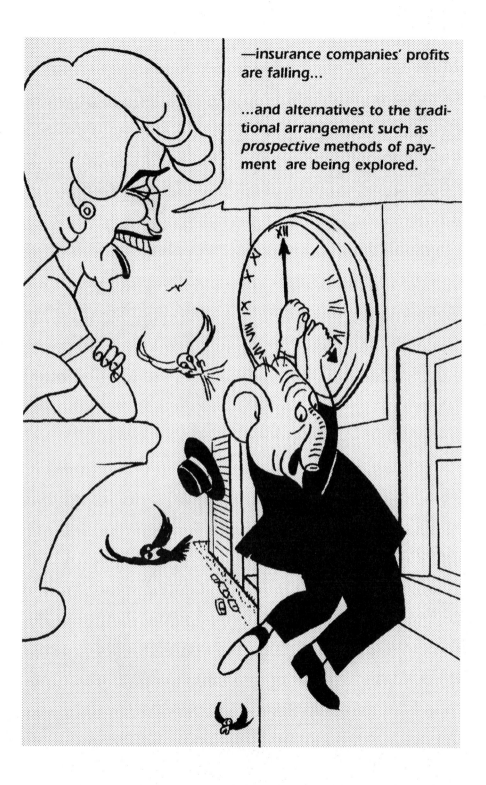

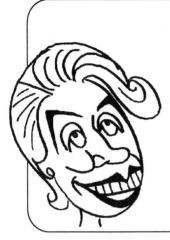

Some thought that the atmosphere of heightened competition between insurance providers and health care providers such as hospitals would result in lowered medical costs to the consumer.

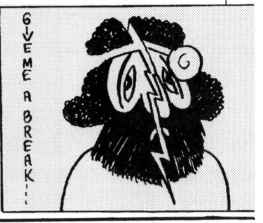

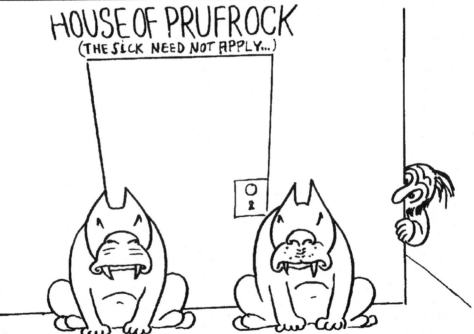

HOUSE OF PRUFROCK
(THE SICK NEED NOT APPLY...)

What's happened instead is that many insurance companies and healthcare provider networks try to weed out or otherwise discourage people with major (= expensive) medical problems from joining them.

Community rating by insurance companies is being increasingly replaced by *experience*-rating: insurance premiums—and even accessibility to insurance—depend on the projected level of an individual's health care needs.

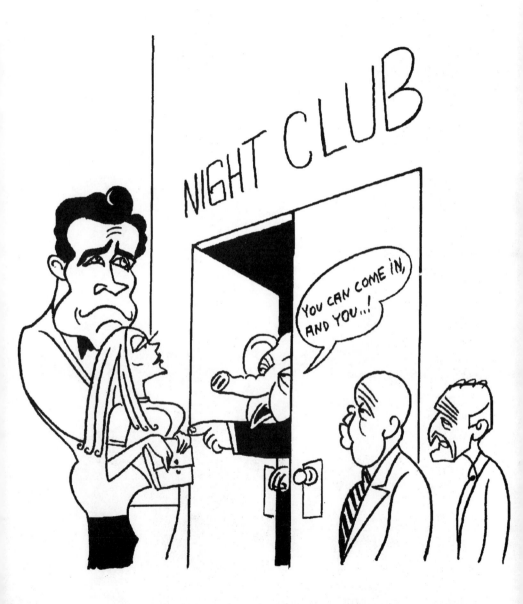

HEALTH CARE COSST$S

Other countries spend less and do better.

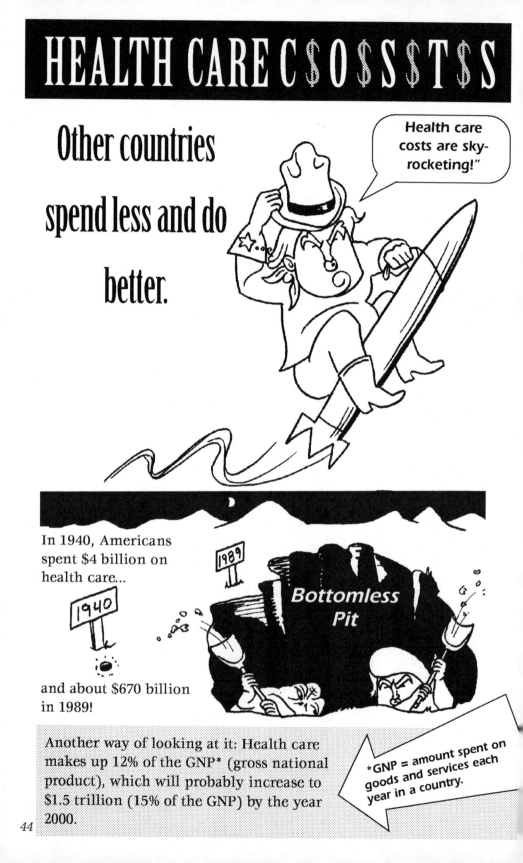

"Health care costs are sky-rocketing!"

In 1940, Americans spent $4 billion on health care...

and about $670 billion in 1989!

Bottomless Pit

Another way of looking at it: Health care makes up 12% of the GNP* (gross national product), which will probably increase to $1.5 trillion (15% of the GNP) by the year 2000.

*GNP = amount spent on goods and services each year in a country.

Countries with national health plans don't suffer from this Runaway Cost Syndrome; in Canada, Great Britain, France, and Germany the size of the health care bite out of the GNP remains the same from year to year...

...unlike the United States, where the percentage of the GNP gobbled up by health care services increases by about 20% each year.

Health care expenditures by the government are on the rise too, growing from about 10% of the budget in 1965 to 30% in 1985.

MEDICARE

EXPENSES IN BILLIONS

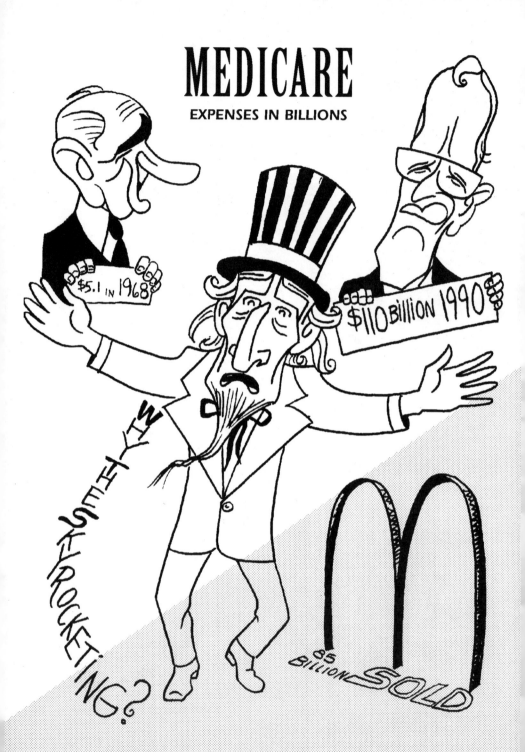

$5.1 IN 1968

$110 BILLION 1990

WHY SKYROCKETING?

$5 BILLION SOLD

Health care is the country's third largest industry.

The average doctor pays over $12,000 each year for malpractice (liability) insurance coverage.

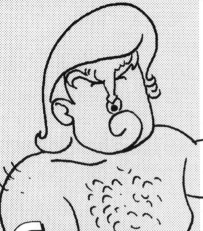

"*A bargain at the price!*"

As the number of malpractice suits (and awards against doctors and hospitals) grows, so does the cost of doctors' liability insurance.

And guess who pays? You and me! Every time my doctor's malpractice insurance goes up, so does his fee!

At least one-third of the doctors in the U.S. have been sued at some point in their careers...with the average award weighing in at about $500,000.

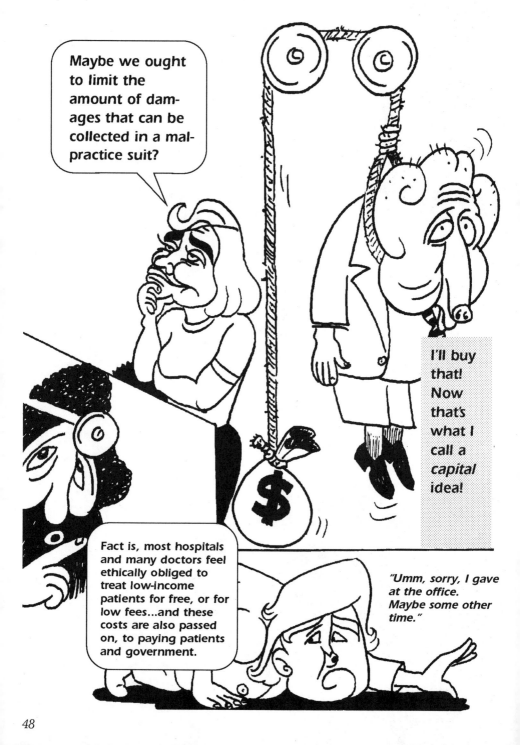

HI-TECH = HIGH FINANCE

When it comes to health care, Americans want the latest and the best.

But they don't want to pay for it! Most U.S. doctors don't think twice about ordering super-expensive tests—even when less costly ones will do.

New technology isn't always good technology.

Case in point: fetal electronic monitoring.

That's right. Nowadays getting born involves having a metal electrode slapped on your poor little scalp.

Even though many obstetricians now feel this is unnecessary...

It's the old "CYA" approach—

"CYA?"

COVER YOUR ASS!

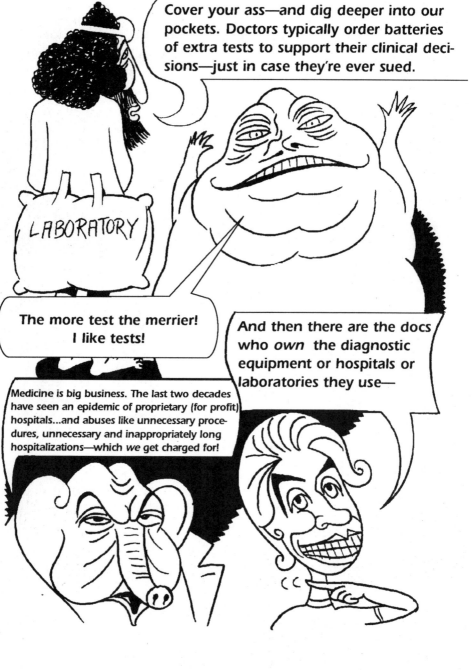

Cover your ass—and dig deeper into our pockets. Doctors typically order batteries of extra tests to support their clinical decisions—just in case they're ever sued.

The more test the merrier! I like tests!

And then there are the docs who *own* the diagnostic equipment or hospitals or laboratories they use—

Medicine is big business. The last two decades have seen an epidemic of proprietary (for profit) hospitals...and abuses like unnecessary procedures, unnecessary and inappropriately long hospitalizations—which *we* get charged for!

LABORATORY

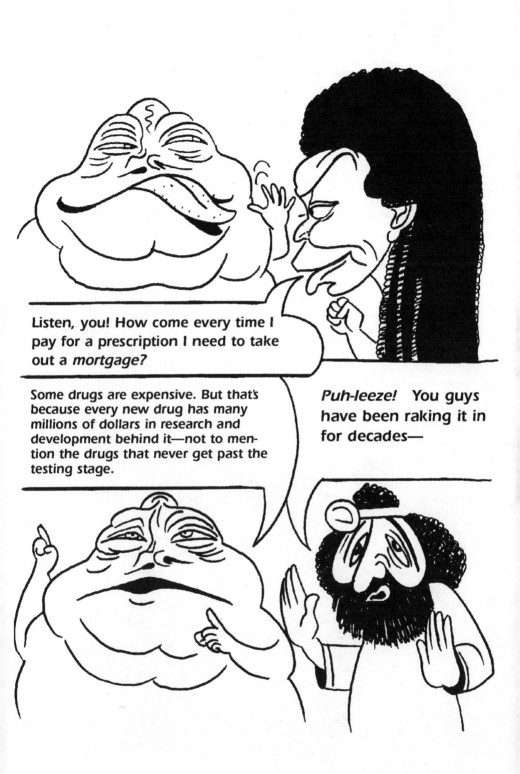

Listen, you! How come every time I pay for a prescription I need to take out a *mortgage?*

Some drugs are expensive. But that's because every new drug has many millions of dollars in research and development behind it—not to mention the drugs that never get past the testing stage.

Puh-leeze! You guys have been raking it in for decades—

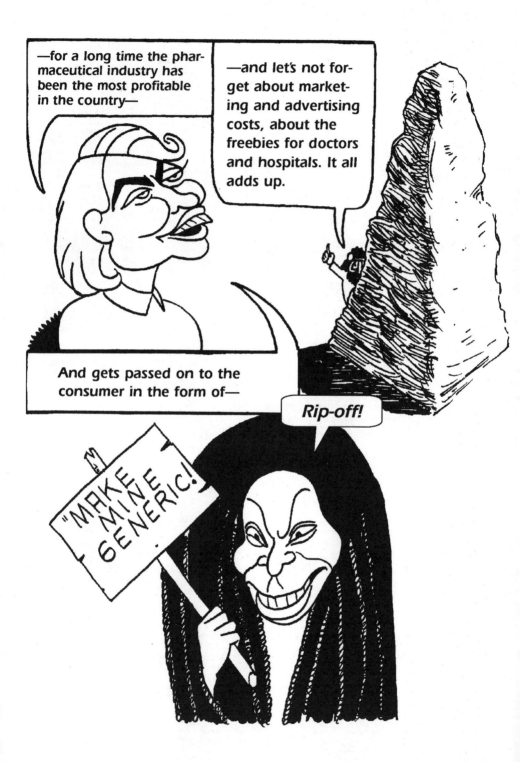

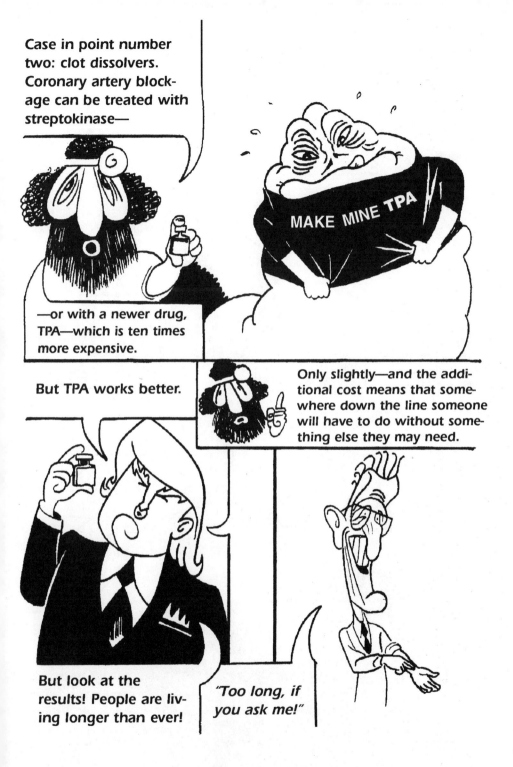

Case in point number two: clot dissolvers. Coronary artery blockage can be treated with streptokinase—

MAKE MINE TPA

—or with a newer drug, TPA—which is ten times more expensive.

But TPA works better.

Only slightly—and the additional cost means that somewhere down the line someone will have to do without something else they may need.

But look at the results! People are living longer than ever!

"Too long, if you ask me!"

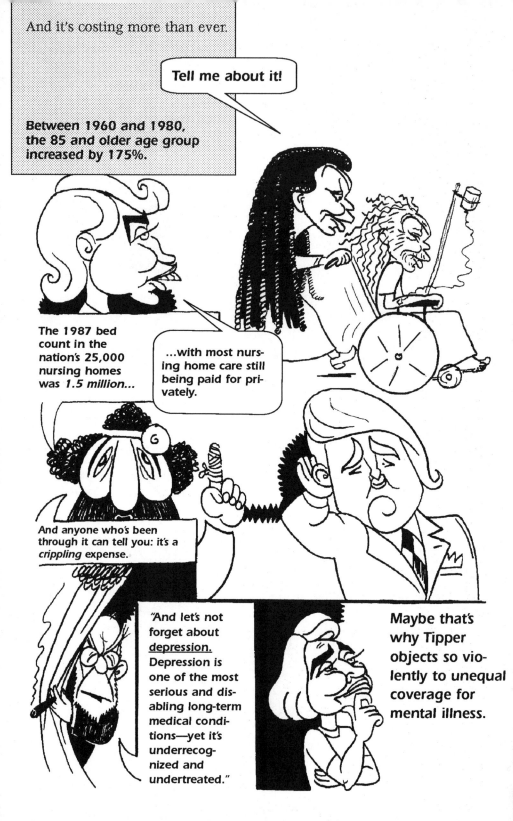

And it's costing more than ever.

Tell me about it!

Between 1960 and 1980, the 85 and older age group increased by 175%.

The 1987 bed count in the nation's 25,000 nursing homes was *1.5 million*...

...with most nursing home care still being paid for privately.

And anyone who's been through it can tell you: it's a *crippling* expense.

"And let's not forget about <u>depression.</u> Depression is one of the most serious and disabling long-term medical conditions—yet it's underrecognized and undertreated."

Maybe that's why Tipper objects so violently to unequal coverage for mental illness.

Between 1970 and 1982, the number of health care providers increased by 57%, while the number of adminstrators increased by 171%.

That's right, administrators: clinic directors, managed care overseers, utilization review technicians, you name it—the cost of supporting all this personnel far exceeds that of a single-payer system...by billions.

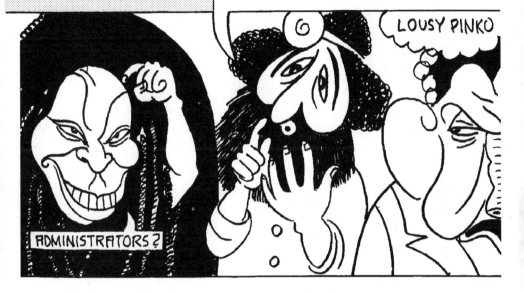

In the U.S., heroic and often awesomely expensive efforts are made to save low birth weight premature babies—while the immunization of children has lower priority.

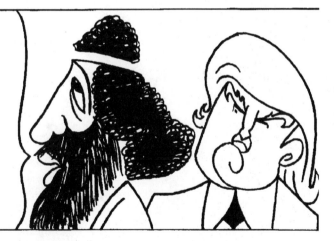

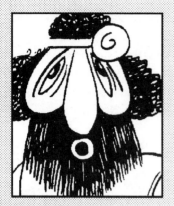

Four out of ten 1 to 4 year olds are not being immunized against mumps, polio, rubella, measles;

the rate of non-immunization is even higher among non-white kids.

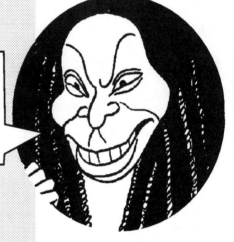

Caesarian sections and coronary artery bypasses are performed twenty-eight times more often here than in some European countries...

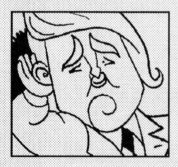

...and although England has only 100 cardiologists, England also has 100 geropsychiatrists.

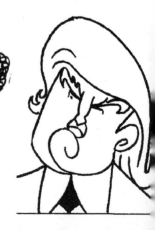

Which is the more important expense? Hi-tech approaches that are available to the few...or standard prevention and treatment for all? Hi-tech for some or waiting in line for many?

Health care policy involves hard *decisions. Not having a national health care policy is also a decision.*

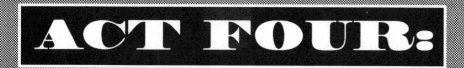

ACT FOUR:

Taking the Horse by the Reins... and Trading it in for a New One

"A recent survey of doctors found that 82% felt that the U.S. health care system was in crisis, and 45% agreed that a complete over-haul was necessary."

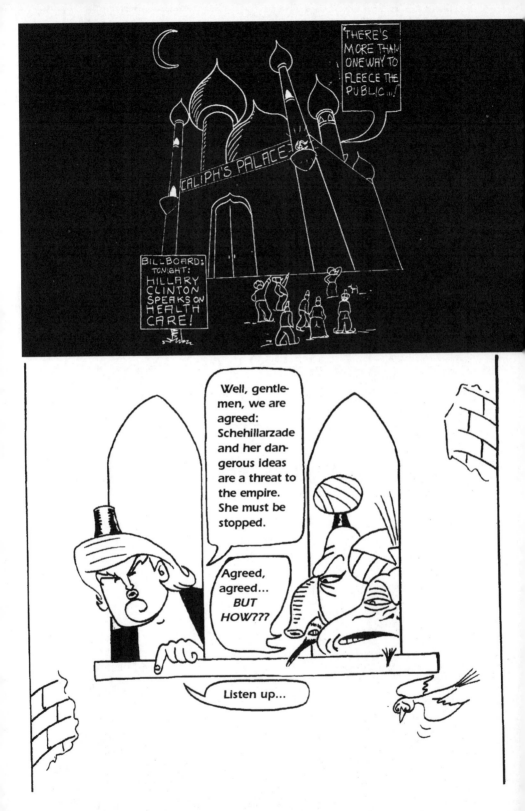

Alternatives to the Traditional Arrangements: a soliloquoy on current insurance plans and practices

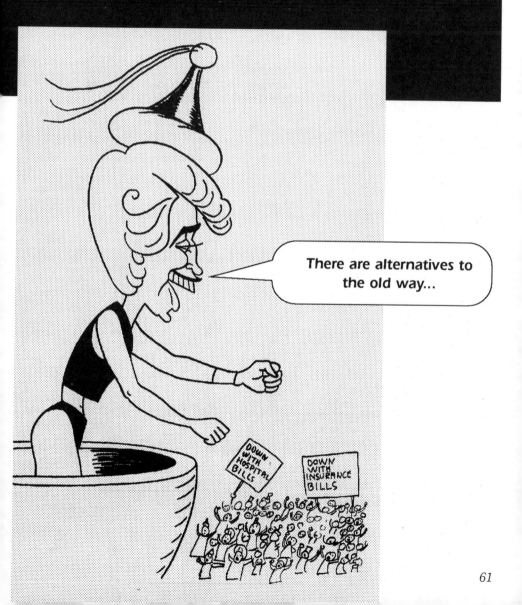

Health Maintenance Organization (HMO):

HMOs (36 million Americans now belong to one or another of these) use a *prospective payment* system.

People enroll in HMOs by paying a monthly or quarterly or annual *pre-payment* (or *capitation*) fee, which covers all health care services used during the period of enroll-ment. Usually there is an additional small fee, something on the order of $5 or $10 dollars, paid by the HMO member each time he or she visits the doctor.

Patients may be assigned to HMO doctors rather than being able to pick them on their own. HMO doctors receive a capitation fee (an annual salary) for each patient they follow in their practice, and the fee is the same regard-less of how often the patient sees the doctor. Since the doctor (or hospital) is no longer receiving a fee for each separate service (or procedure or day of hospitalization) rendered, doctors in HMOs streamline or offer the most cost- or labor-effective treatments.

APPLY HERE FOR HMO

EXIT

MD

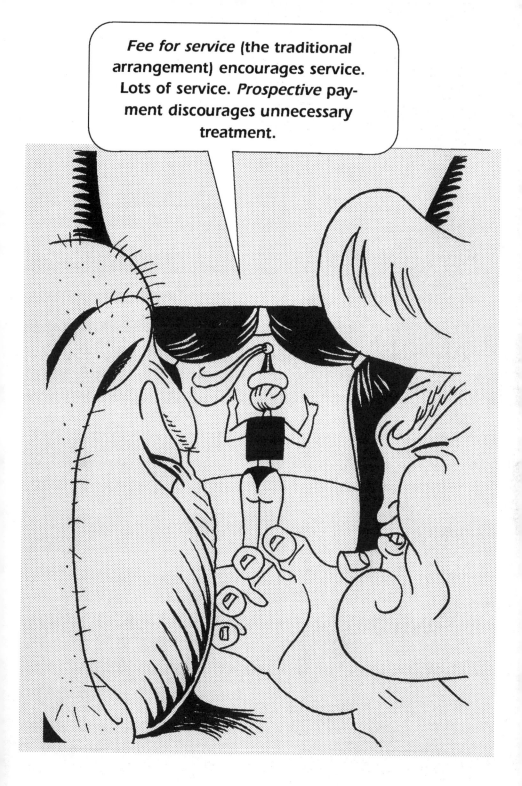

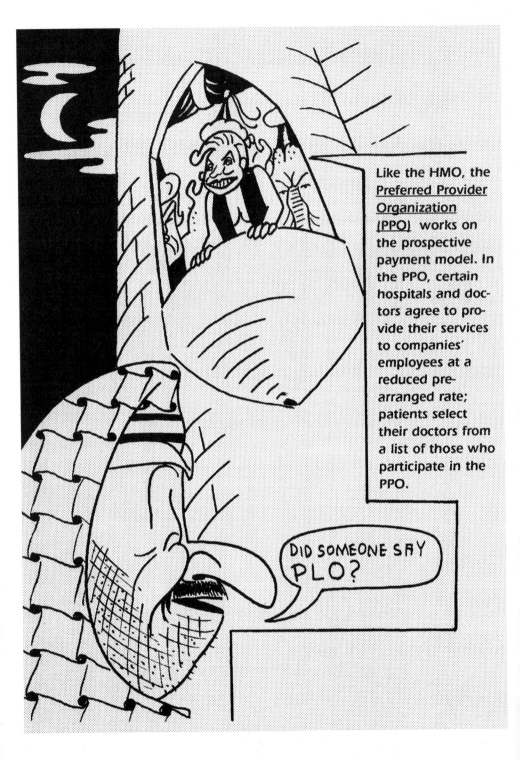

Like the HMO, the Preferred Provider Organization (PPO) works on the prospective payment model. In the PPO, certain hospitals and doctors agree to provide their services to companies' employees at a reduced pre-arranged rate; patients select their doctors from a list of those who participate in the PPO.

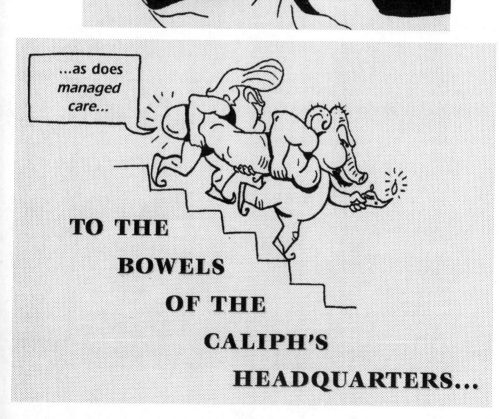

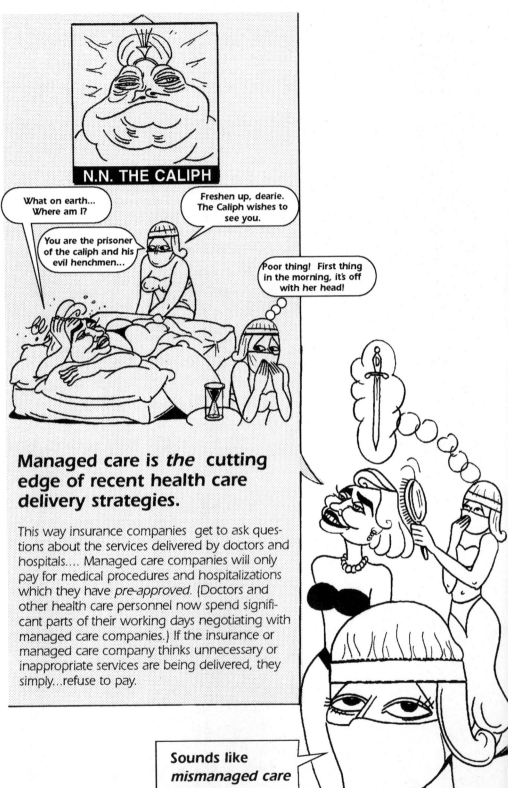

Managed care is *the* cutting edge of recent health care delivery strategies.

This way insurance companies get to ask questions about the services delivered by doctors and hospitals.... Managed care companies will only pay for medical procedures and hospitalizations which they have *pre-approved*. (Doctors and other health care personnel now spend significant parts of their working days negotiating with managed care companies.) If the insurance or managed care company thinks unnecessary or inappropriate services are being delivered, they simply...refuse to pay.

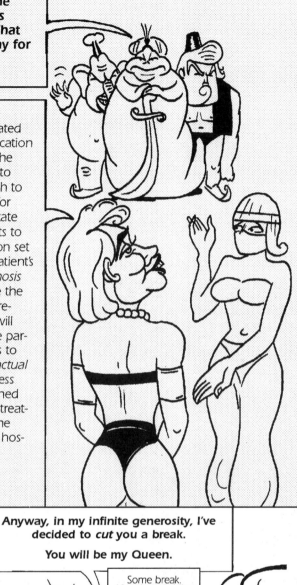

Ha ha! If it isn't the lovely but helpless Schehillarzade. What do you have to say for yourself?

DRGs (Diagnosis Related Groups) are a classification system adopted by the federal government to determine how much to reimburse hospitals for Medicare patients. State and federal payments to hospitals are based on set fees related to the patient's diagnosis (i.e., *diagnosis related group*.) Since the hospital knows before-hand how much it will receive based on the particular DRG, it stands to make money if the *actual* cost of treatment is less than the predetermined amount. Likewise, if treatment costs exceed the DRG allowance, the hospital loses money.

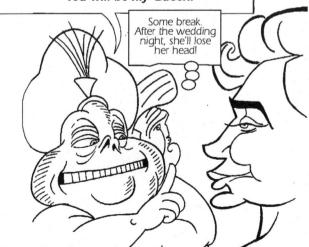

Anyway, in my infinite generosity, I've decided to *cut* you a break.

You will be my Queen.

Some break. After the wedding night, she'll lose her head!

RBRVS (Resource-Based Relative Value Scale) is a system designed to help third-party payers determine how much to reimburse doctors. Health care services and providers are rated for things like the length of the procedure, the expense of overhead, the cost of running a doctor's office, and the cost of the doctor's training.

Er, don't we have pressing affairs of state...?

That's right. I'll see you in the bridal suite, dearie.

PSROs (Professional Standards Review Organization) was created by the government to review quality of health care paid for with federal funds. These have also been set up on a local basis by medical associations for monitoring of practice standards of physicians.

PROs (Peer Review Organization) replaced PSROs as the federal system that reviews hospital costs to Medicare.

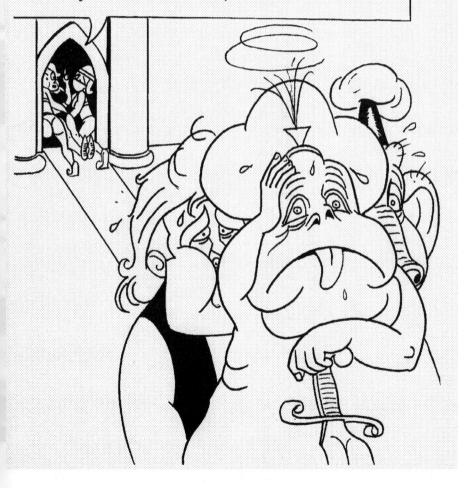

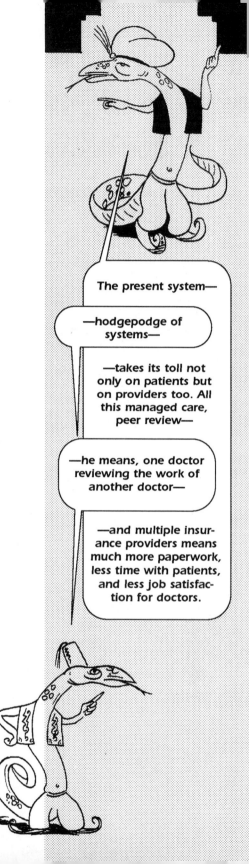

The present system—

—hodgepodge of systems—

—takes its toll not only on patients but on providers too. All this managed care, peer review—

—he means, one doctor reviewing the work of another doctor—

—and multiple insurance providers means much more paperwork, less time with patients, and less job satisfaction for doctors.

Almost half of doctors over age 35 stated in a recent survey that they would not suggest medicine as a career choice. And compared with a survey taken in 1971, more doctors in 1992 felt that national health insurance would actually improve care by reaching more patients. A recent survey of doctors found that 82% felt the U.S. health care system was in crisis, and 45% agreed that a complete overhaul was necessary. And polls tell us that people distrust insurance companies even more than they do the government.

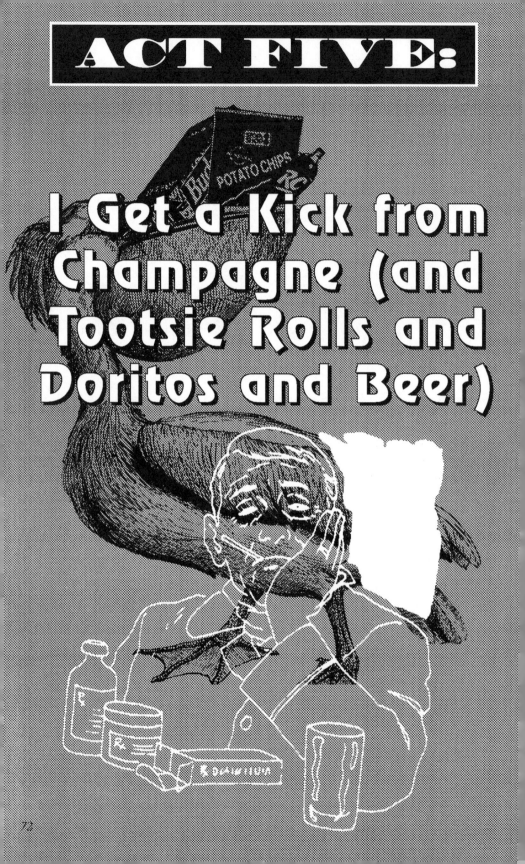

ACT FIVE:

I Get a Kick from Champagne (and Tootsie Rolls and Doritos and Beer)

"Only 0.3% of our national health budget goes for prevention. Major improvements in U.S. life expectancy...are mostly due to *preventive* efforts such as progress in social factors like diet and housing conditions."

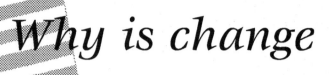

Why is change

It's got a lot to
do with lifestyle.

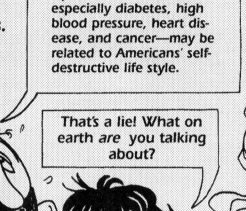

Up to 70% of all illness—
especially diabetes, high
blood pressure, heart disease, and cancer—may be
related to Americans' self-
destructive life style.

That's a lie! What on
earth *are* you talking
about?

AN OUNCE OF PREVENTION...

so slow to come?

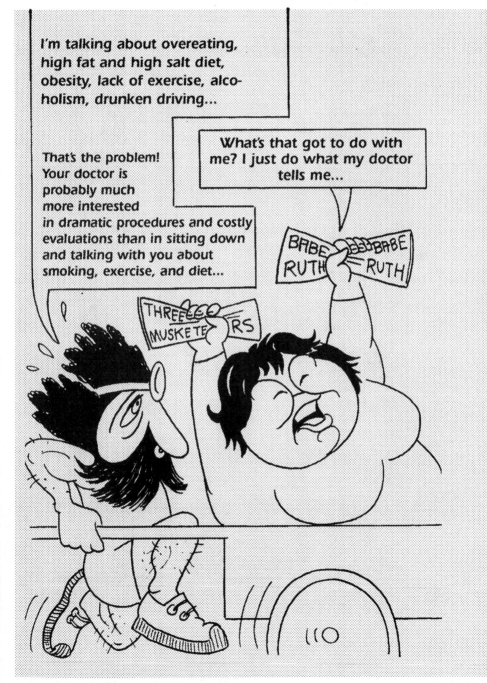

Only 0.3% of our national health budget goes for prevention. Major improvements in U.S. life expectancy and infant mortality over the past thirty or more years are mostly due to *preventive* efforts such as prenatal care and vaccination and to progress in social factors like diet and housing conditions. Preventive efforts aimed at eliminating or reducing environmental toxins from industry would also have an enormous impact on the health of Americans.

With improved life expectancy, chronic medical conditions predominate... but the current system does little to provide for nursing homes and other extended health care systems.

Van Winkle NURSING HOME
CASH ONLY — PLEASE

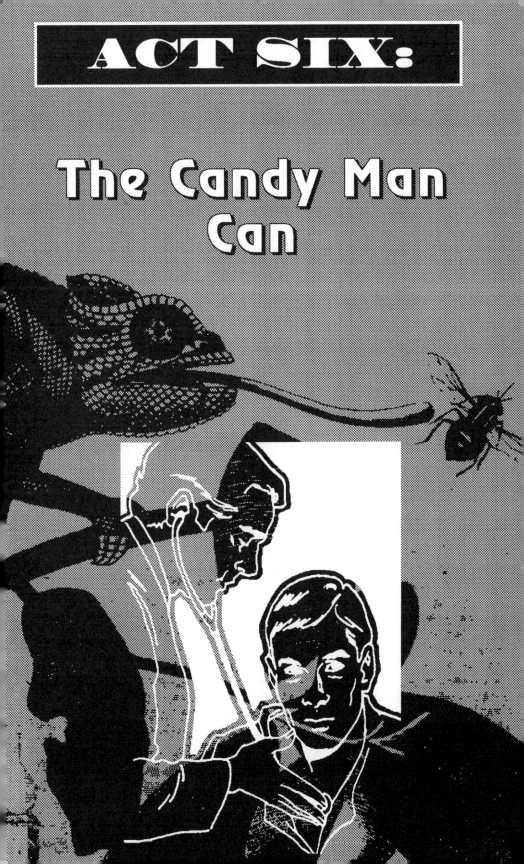

"People don't realize the enormous expense involved in producing a new drug. And how these mind-boggling costs get passed along to YOU!!!"

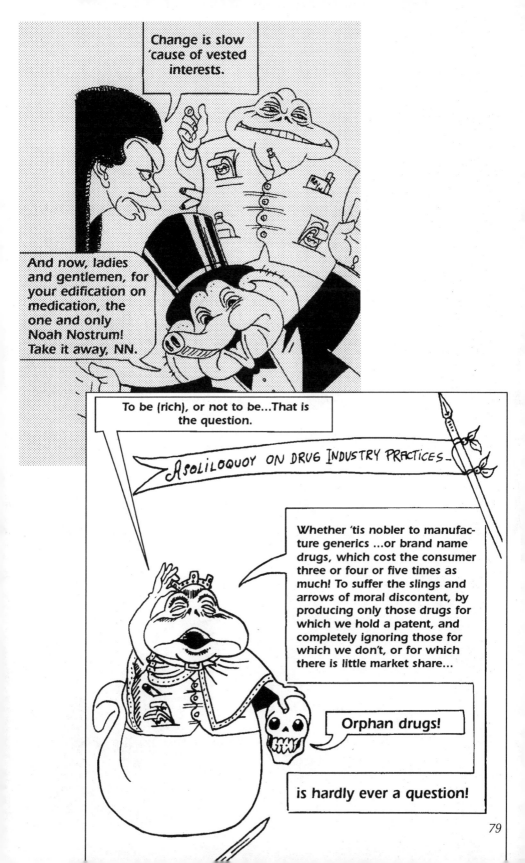

79

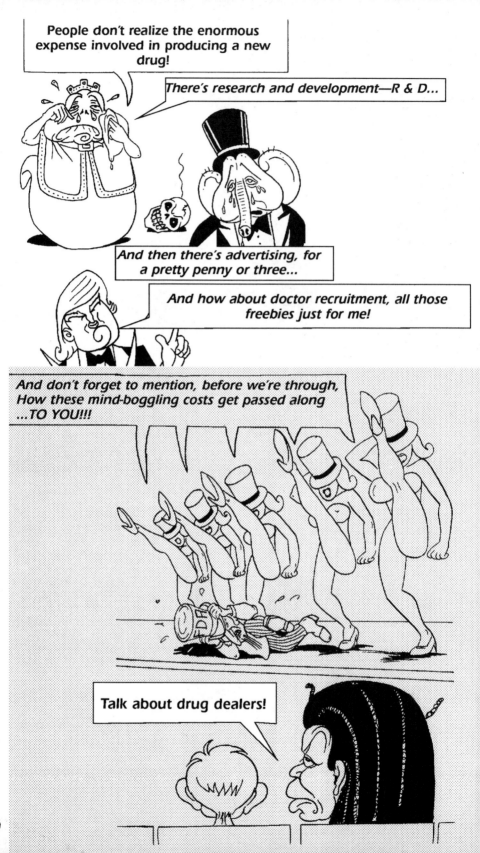

ACT SEVEN:

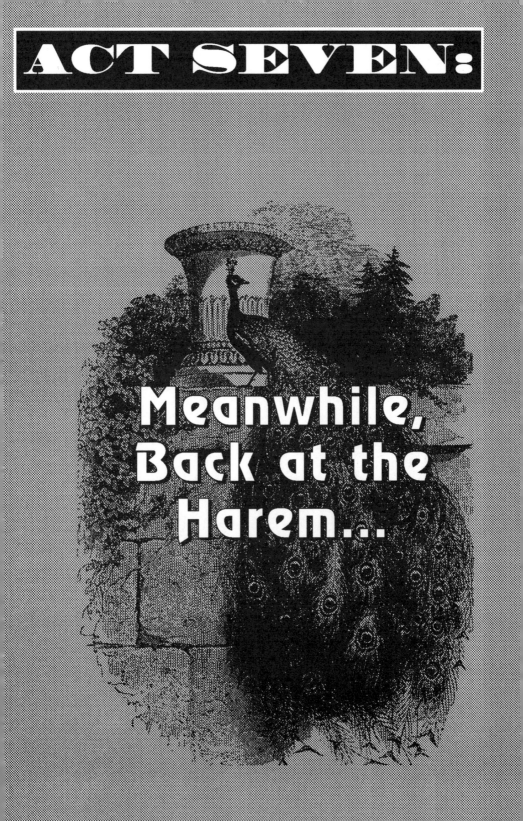

Meanwhile,
Back at the
Harem...

"Countries with national health care, like Canada and Great Britain, don't pass major portions of medical costs on to patients; yet these countries have lower overall medical costs than the U.S."

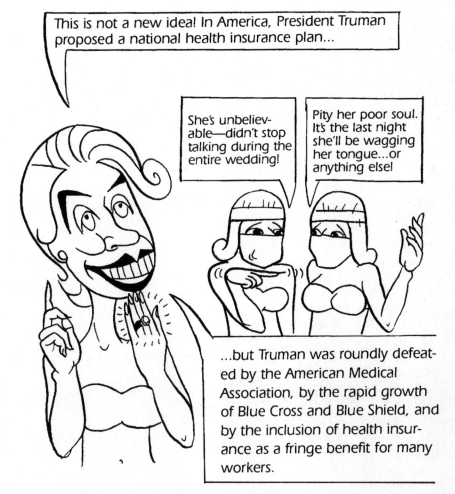

This is not a new idea! In America, President Truman proposed a national health insurance plan...

She's unbelievable—didn't stop talking during the entire wedding!

Pity her poor soul. It's the last night she'll be wagging her tongue...or anything else!

...but Truman was roundly defeated by the American Medical Association, by the rapid growth of Blue Cross and Blue Shield, and by the inclusion of health insurance as a fringe benefit for many workers.

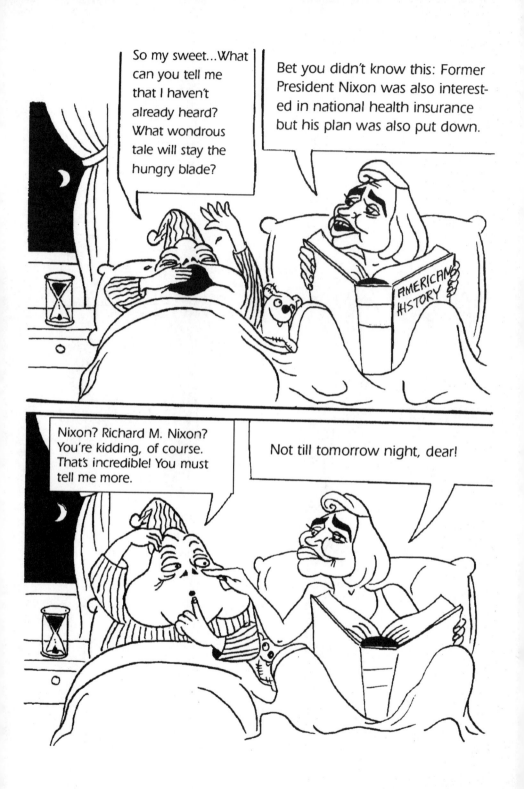

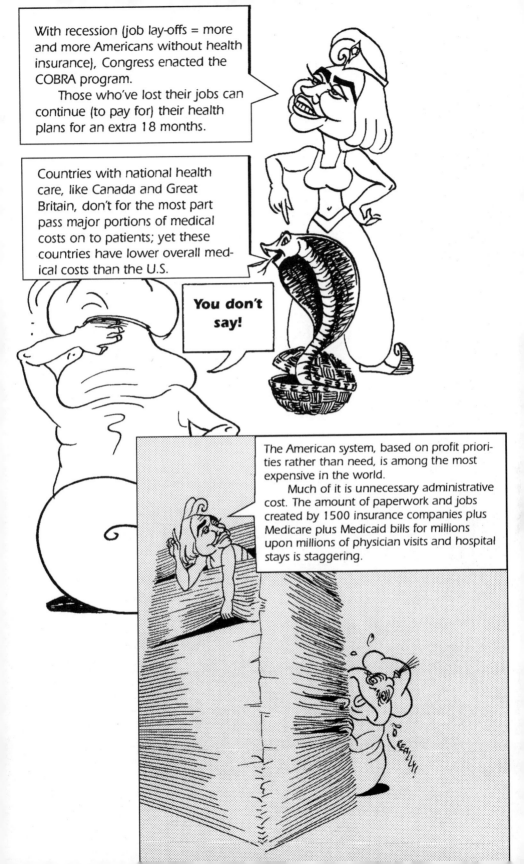

With recession (job lay-offs = more and more Americans without health insurance), Congress enacted the COBRA program.

Those who've lost their jobs can continue (to pay for) their health plans for an extra 18 months.

Countries with national health care, like Canada and Great Britain, don't for the most part pass major portions of medical costs on to patients; yet these countries have lower overall medical costs than the U.S.

You don't say!

The American system, based on profit priorities rather than need, is among the most expensive in the world.

Much of it is unnecessary administrative cost. The amount of paperwork and jobs created by 1500 insurance companies plus Medicare plus Medicaid bills for millions upon millions of physician visits and hospital stays is staggering.

Plus the American system is very, very inefficient— poor people, those without insurance, very often rely for their medical care on emergency rooms...where they sometimes must wait hours and days for hospital admission. The cost of this charity care is passed along to those who pay for insurance, either privately or through taxes (cost shifting). A hidden cost of the uninsured poor relying on emergency rooms is that they have only minimal exposure to follow-up or continued care.

Preventive medicine?

Exactly...so poor people wouldn't have to seek treatment for problems that are already full-blown, serious, and therefore expensive.

I see your point...

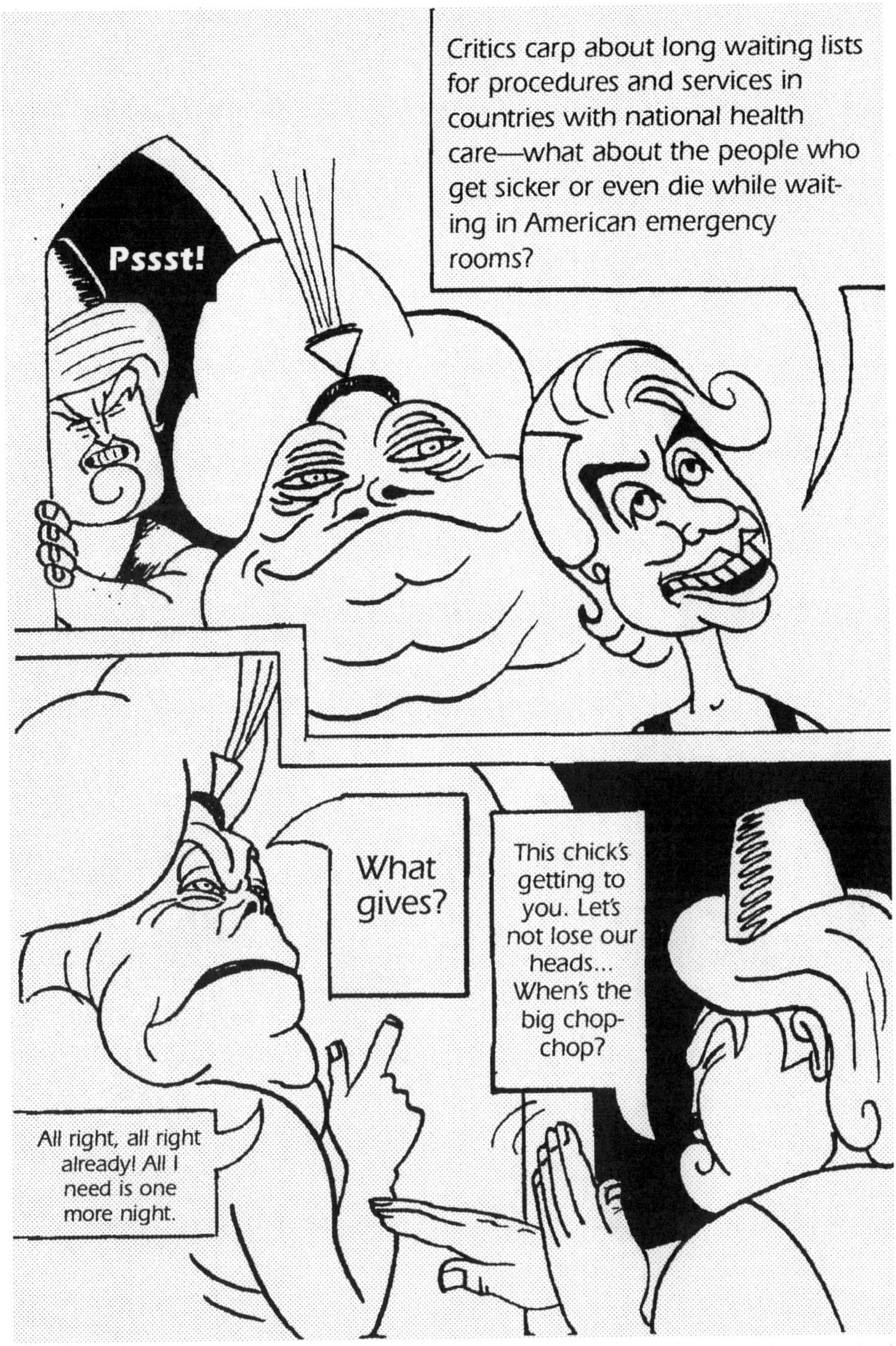
Critics carp about long waiting lists for procedures and services in countries with national health care—what about the people who get sicker or even die while waiting in American emergency rooms?
Pssst!
What gives?
This chick's getting to you. Let's not lose our heads... When's the big chop-chop?
All right, all right already! All I need is one more night.

And then there's AIDS. There's no way that people with AIDS can afford proper treatment under the present system.

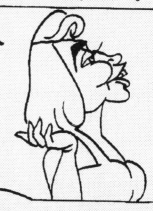

My viziers are right. Enough with the high-minded talk. I'm gonna hand her her head at dawn.

In America, keeping up the *appearance* of a free market, for-profit health care system (which, in fact, is significantly supported by state and federal money and excludes a large part of the population from the health care they need) is literally a crippling expense. It is highly likely that the savings resulting from the elimination of such unnecessary expenses *could cover that portion of the U.S. population that is presently uninsured....*

Well, my dear, anything else before we turn in?

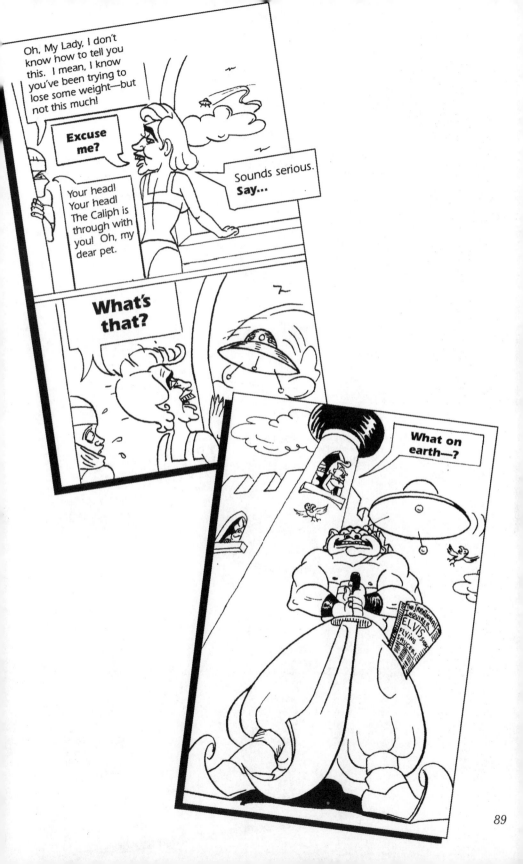

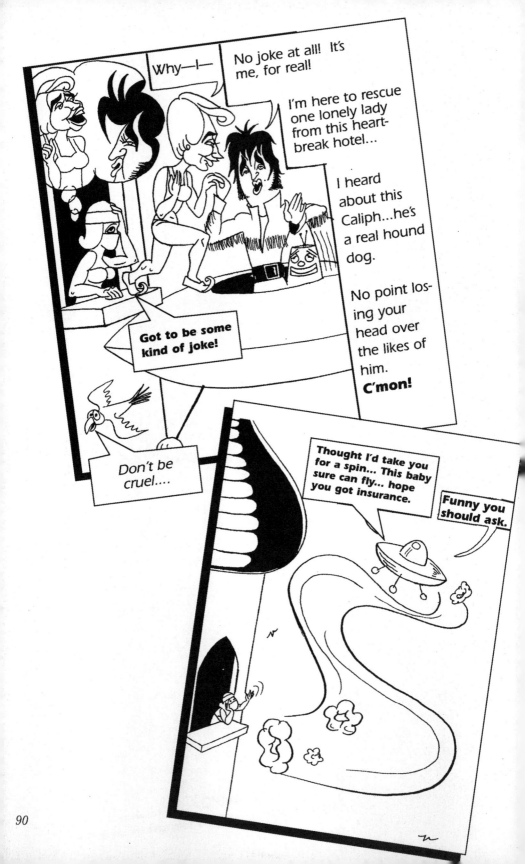

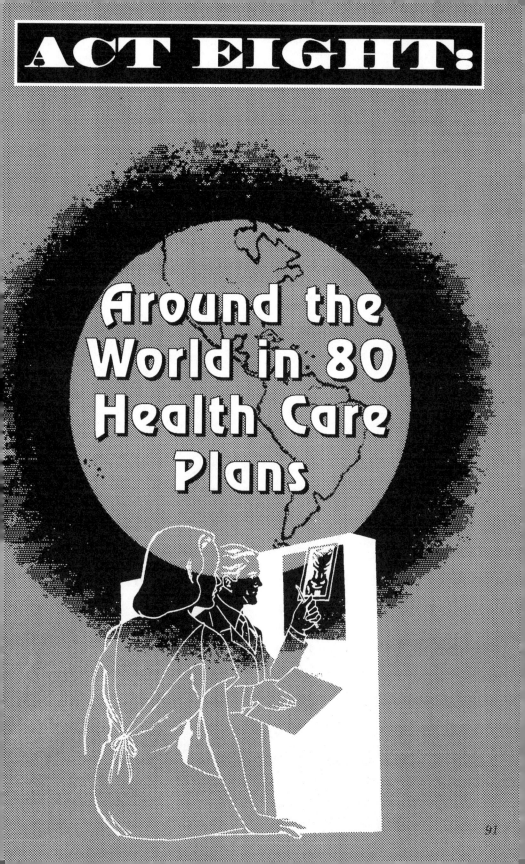

ACT EIGHT:

Around the World in 80 Health Care Plans

Report of United States General Accounting Office (1991):

"...if the universal coverage and single-payer features of the Canadian system were applied in the United States, the savings in administrative costs alone would be more than enough to finance insurance coverage for the millions of Americans who are currently uninsured."

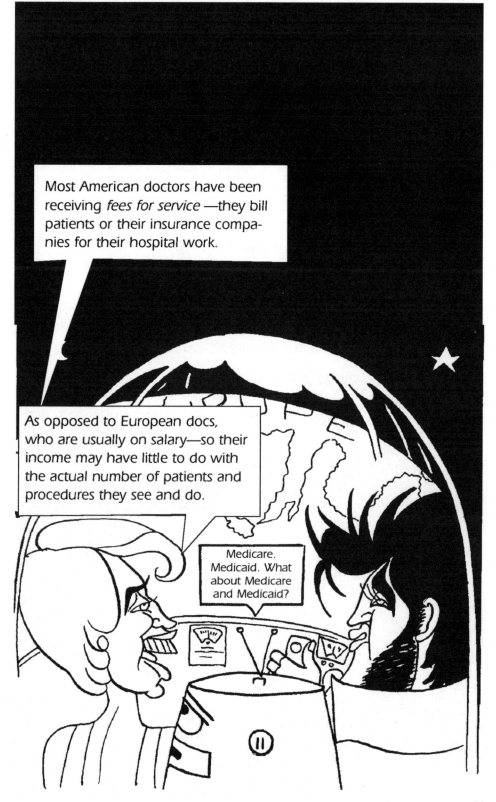

Fewer and fewer American doctors participate in governmentally funded programs, because the fees are so low. But it's possible that these same doctors might favor a national Medicare/Medicaid-type plan that offered more appropriate fees, especially since a large part of doctors' and hospitals' services are provided free now to poor people.

Countries with national health plans—Canada, Great Britain, Germany, among others—use *global budgeting,* which is a form of prospective payment. It's the one centralized element that is critical and allows all the other strategies to work. Global budgeting creates an annual upper limit on how much can be spent on the state, province, or national level. Each of these countries spends comparatively less on health care than the U.S.—yet the quality is said to be equivalent.

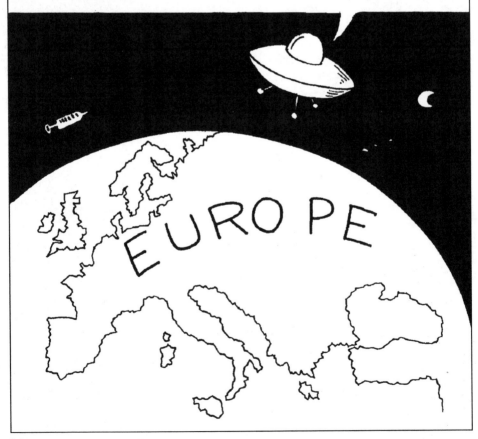

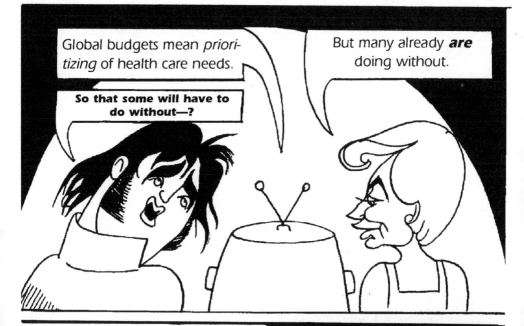

So that some will have to do without—?

Global budgets mean *prioritizing* of health care needs.

But many already **are** doing without.

Canada's *National Health Insurance* (NHI) plan, decades in the planning but finally set up in 1971, is often held up as a model.

It features:
- Financing from both the federal and the provincial governments. Government sets an annual limit on medical costs; if these are exceeded, then there is an overall reduction of reimbursement.

- Universal coverage, with no patient co-payments.

- Fee-for-service system, with fees worked out province by province. Doctors who participate in NHI system cannot also have private patients.

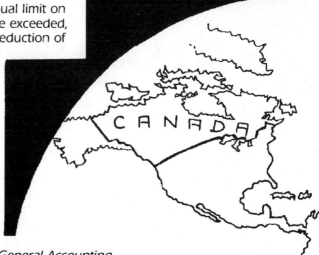

Report of United States General Accounting Office (1991): "...if the universal coverage and single-payer features of the Canadian system were applied in the United States, the savings in administrative costs alone would be more than enough to finance insurance coverage for the millions of Americans who are currently uninsured."

...although some see the Canadian system as approaching a crisis, since costs each year are exceeding the maximum set rate.

95

Of course, China, Cuba, and former USSR are the only *truly* nationalized health care systems, with the government both owning and paying for all health care delivery systems.

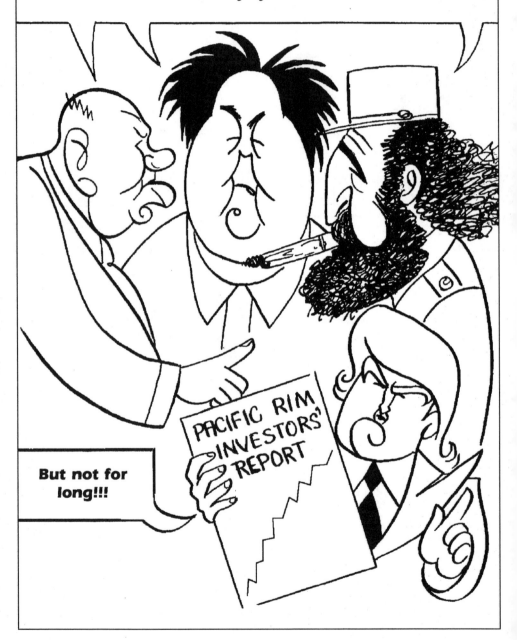

Brits get universal health coverage through their *National Health Service*: The government owns most of the hospitals and pays salaries to hospital doctors. Other doctors' services are contracted for by the government, which reimburses them a fixed amount for each patient they see in their practice annually; additional income is received from administering vaccinations and preventive exams. Patients can choose which doctor they wish to see. The British NHS also makes some allowances for those who wish to access private hospital beds or private care for certain operations. All patients must register with a general practitioner; the G.P. then decides who needs to see a specialist.

IRELAND

ENGLAND

A quick flick of the throttle...and we're an ocean away!

I compute problems.

But the British spend only a fraction of what Americans do on health care!

There *are* problems. Problems such as waiting lists and rationing of hi-tech procedures like heart surgery.

Hold on...we're heading South.

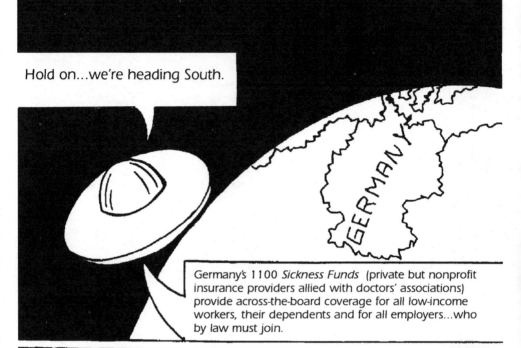

Germany's 1100 *Sickness Funds* (private but nonprofit insurance providers allied with doctors' associations) provide across-the-board coverage for all low-income workers, their dependents and for all employers...who by law must join.

"Take two *bratwurszt* and call me in the morning!"

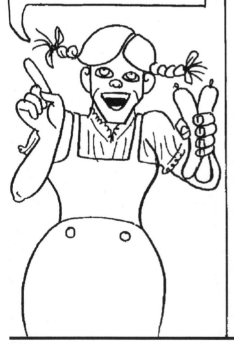

Insurance costs are split down the middle by workers and employers. (Unemployed persons and retirees are covered through a separate arrangement.) Sickness funds use global budgeting. Worker/employer premiums cannot rise faster than workers' incomes do; sickness fund managers use these figures to work out annual payment rates for providers.

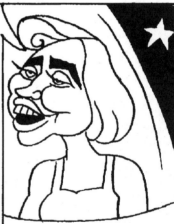

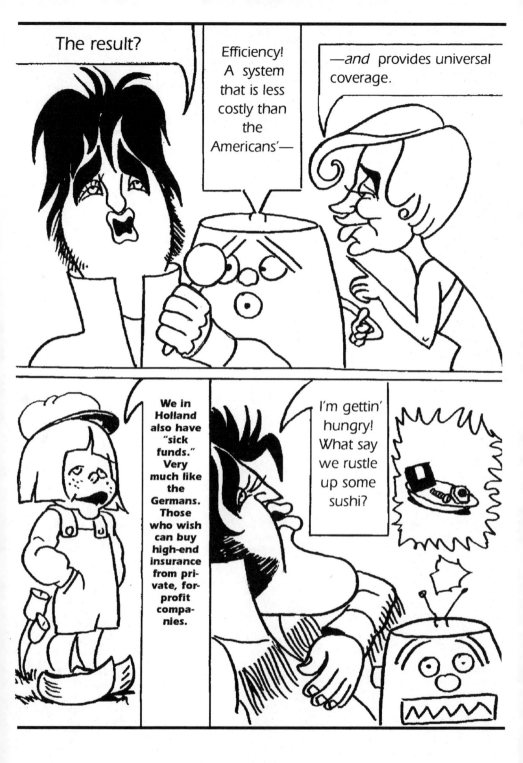

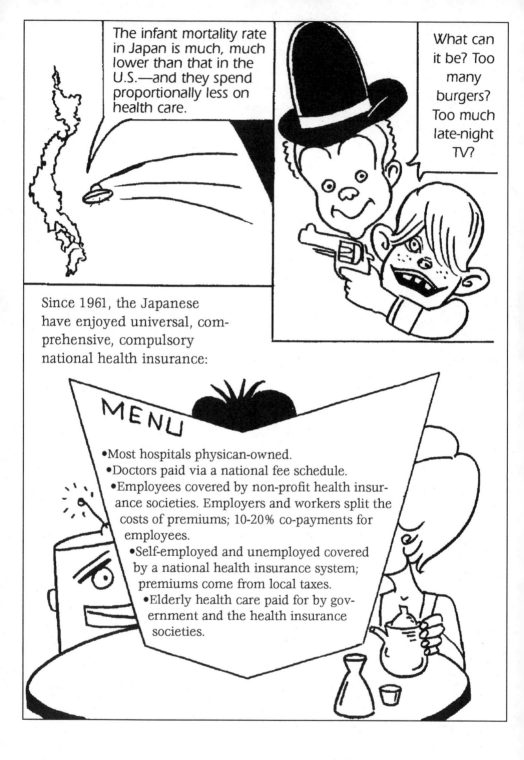

The infant mortality rate in Japan is much, much lower than that in the U.S.—and they spend proportionally less on health care.

What can it be? Too many burgers? Too much late-night TV?

Since 1961, the Japanese have enjoyed universal, comprehensive, compulsory national health insurance:

MENU

• Most hospitals physican-owned.
• Doctors paid via a national fee schedule.
• Employees covered by non-profit health insurance societies. Employers and workers split the costs of premiums; 10-20% co-payments for employees.
• Self-employed and unemployed covered by a national health insurance system; premiums come from local taxes.
• Elderly health care paid for by government and the health insurance societies.

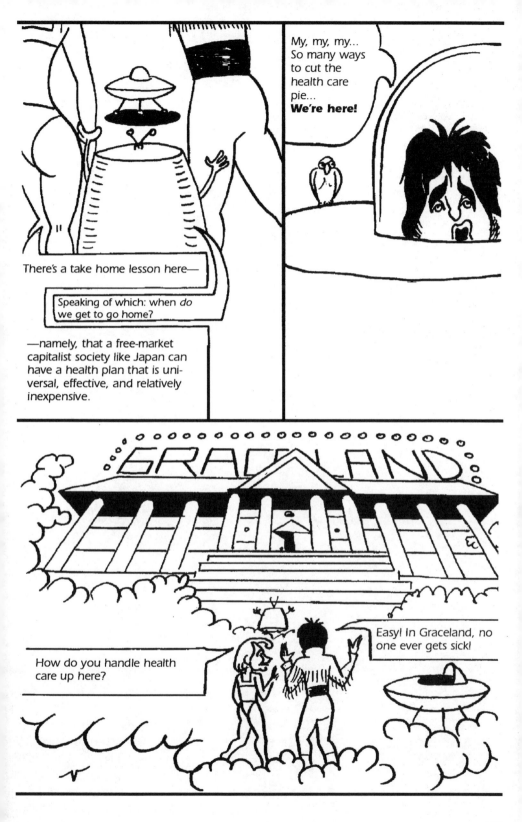

There's a take home lesson here—

Speaking of which: when *do* we get to go home?

—namely, that a free-market capitalist society like Japan can have a health plan that is universal, effective, and relatively inexpensive.

My, my, my... So many ways to cut the health care pie... **We're here!**

How do you handle health care up here?

Easy! In Graceland, no one ever gets sick!

ACT NINE:

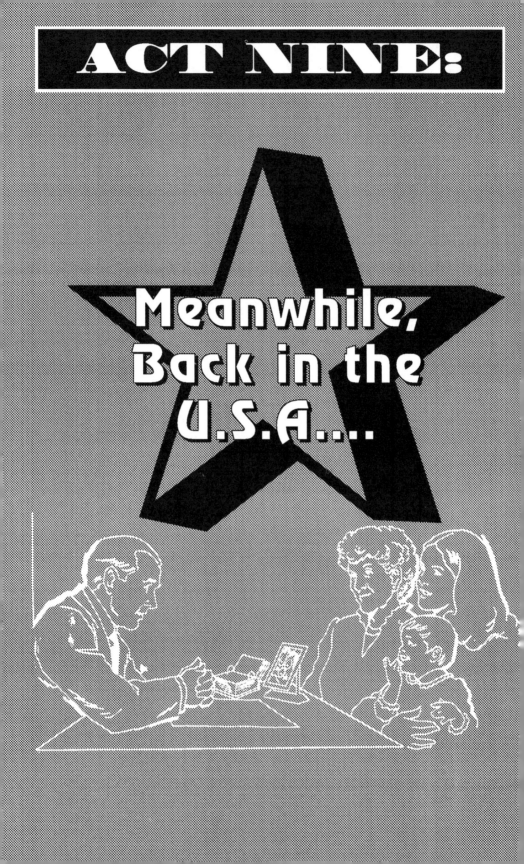

Meanwhile, Back in the U.S.A....

"What we're proposing is this:

There'd be three options:
A low-cost HMO-type plan;
A high-end fee-for-service
plan;
And a combination plan,
costing somewhere in
between.
Prescription drugs, dental
care for children, and
extended care such as nursing homes and rehab centers
would be covered to a certain
extent as well."

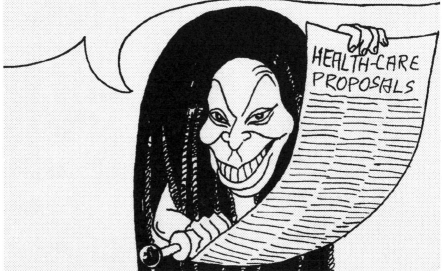

People are practically up in arms.

People keep jobs they hate, because change of job could mean loss of insurance.

Just about *everyone's* dissatisfied—consumers and providers alike.

But not for lack of suggestions!

Proprosals currently on the table:

There's the Physicians for a National Health Plan and their National Health Plan; Senator Kerry's "Health USA"; "Pay or Play" (employers pay for workers' health insurance or pay a tax that goes toward a government-run insurance plan); the Rockefeller-Pepper Commission's Plan; Alain Enthoven's "Managed Competition"; the American Medical Association's "Health Access America" plan; schemes that would make private insurance more affordable via enforced community rating and substantial tax deductions for the self-employed; and if that's not enough, get this:

The prestigious *New England Journal of Medicine* and more recently the American College of Surgeons have come out in favor of a single payer system that would eliminate the insurance middlemen...

Good Grief!

I say we keep it simple!

Every American would be required to have health insurance. Employers would pay at least 80% of this, including premiums for employees' dependents. Workers would contribute 20%, plus any deductibles or co-payments. The self- and un-employed would also be required to buy tax-deductible insurance; some might qualify for government subsidies as well.

What we proposed was this.

There were three options: a low cost HMO-type plan; a high-end fee-for-service plan; and a combination plan, costing somewhere in between. Consumers would be encouraged to join HMOs because of their low cost.

Prescription drugs, dental care for children, and extended care such as nursing homes and rehab centers would be covered to a certain extent as well.

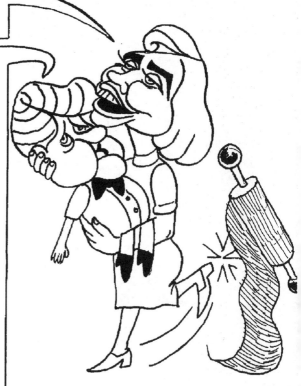

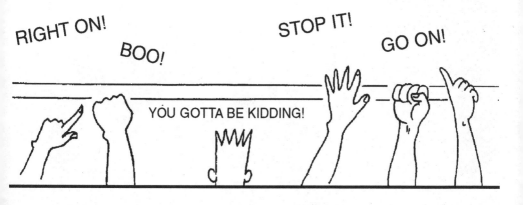

RIGHT ON!

BOO!

STOP IT!

GO ON!

YOU GOTTA BE KIDDING!

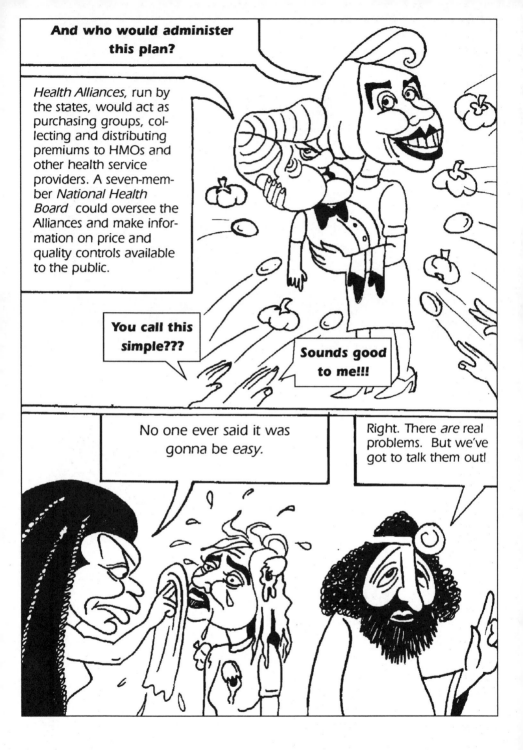

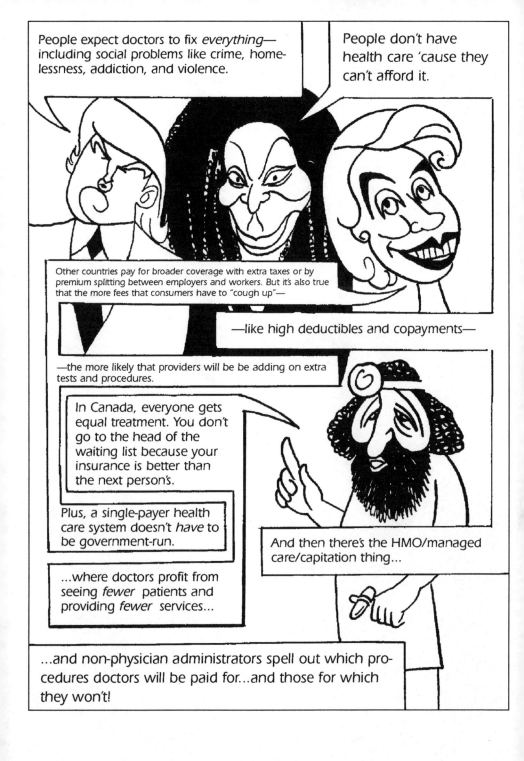

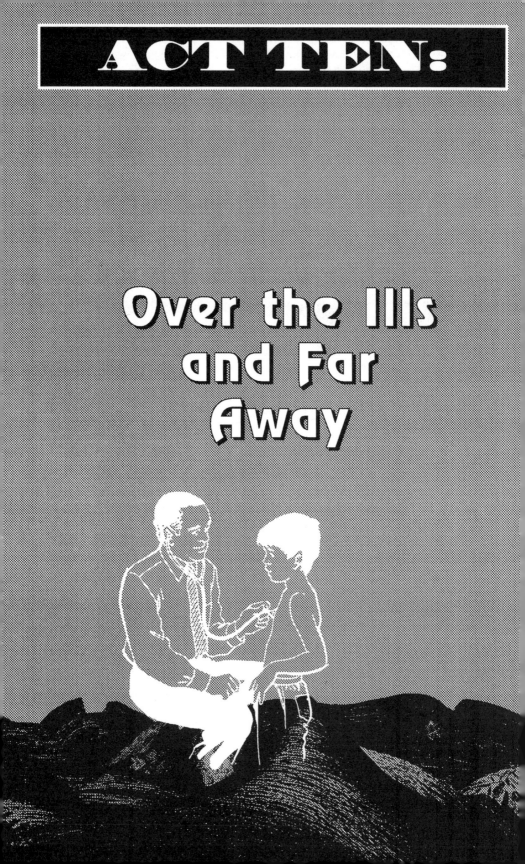

ACT TEN:

Over the Ills and Far Away

"Security is what this debate is all about. Everyone would get a health security card, which would guarantee all Americans access to a comprehensive package of benefits, no matter where they work, where they live, and whether or not they've ever been sick before."

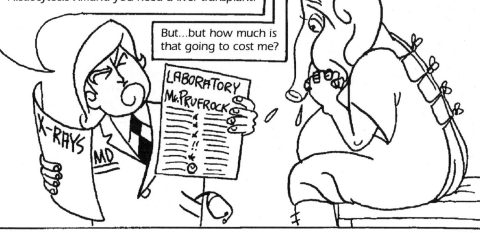

Tsk, tsk. Hmm.

Got some bad news for you, Poiney... You're sick.

What *is* it?

Double—no, let's make that *triple*—sick. Let's see...Gaucher's disease... Histiocytosis X...and you need a liver transplant.

But...but how much is that going to cost me?

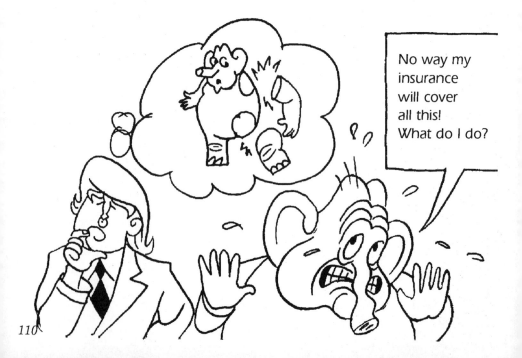

No way my insurance will cover all this! What do I do?

110

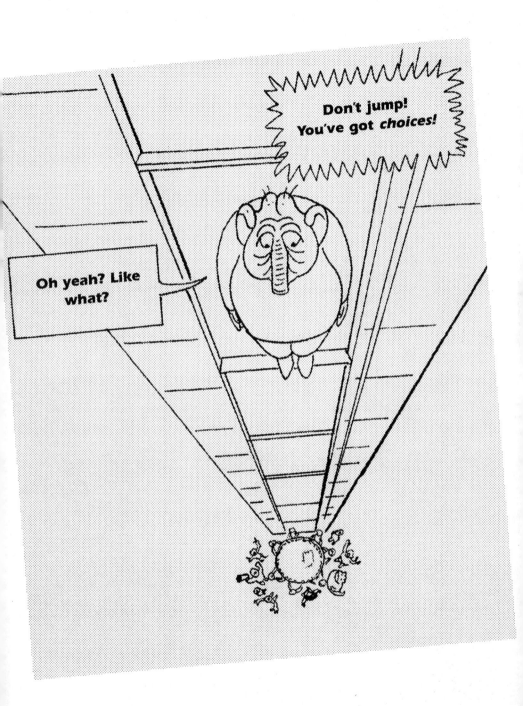

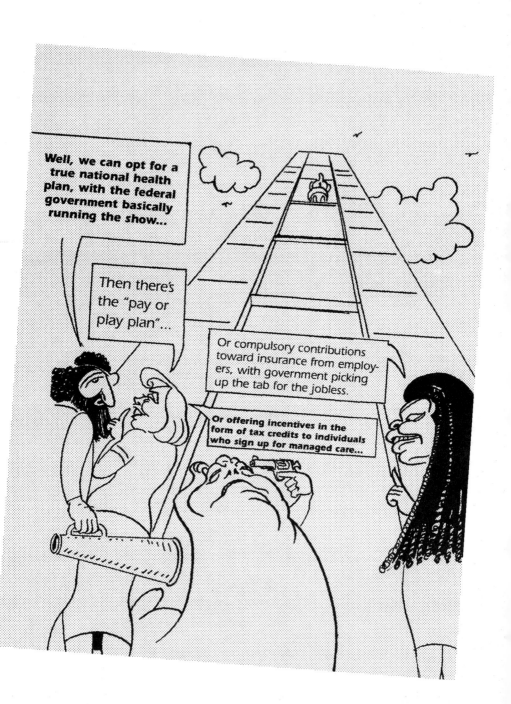

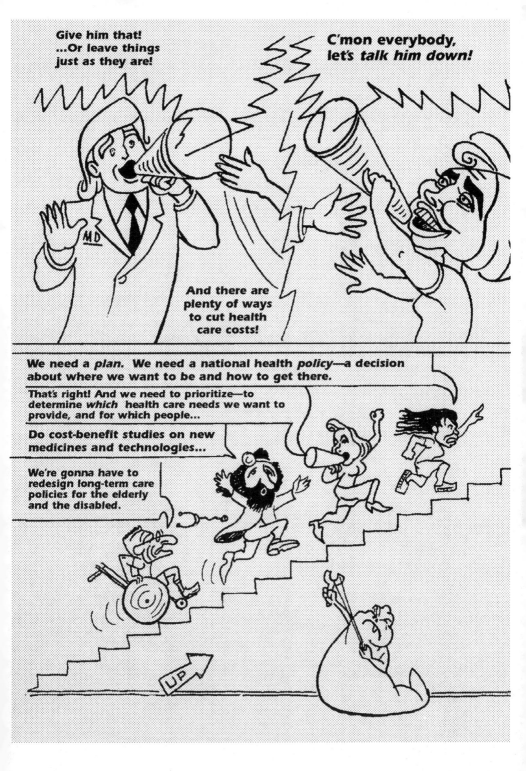

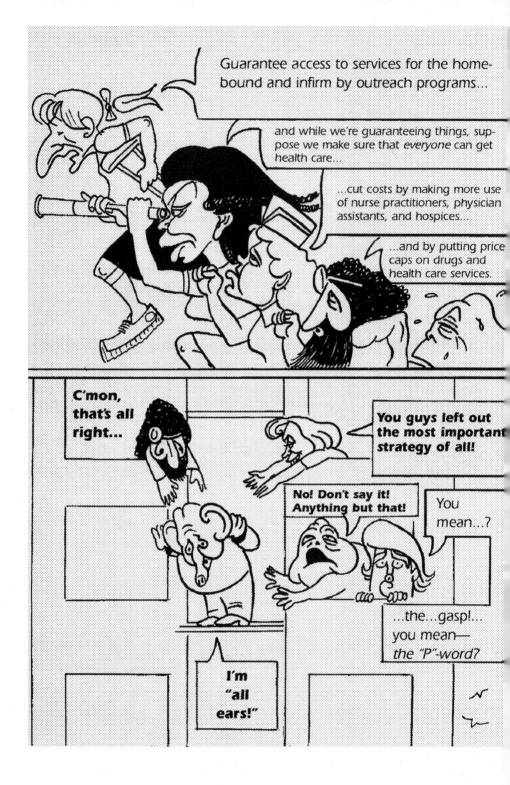

That's right, pal—

—PREVENTION!
The healthier we are, the less likely we'll get sick! We need a *wellness* approach to health, with widely available screening and preventive and educational services.

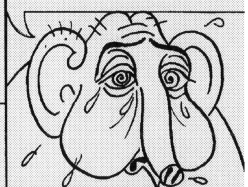

You mean...sob....
No more Cuban cigars?
Cutting down on the
booze? And I might actually
have to...*exercise?*

Sure that'd save billions in insurance payments for doctors and drugs and hospitals...but as for me, in my own life—NO CAN DO!!! Bye, bye, cruel world!

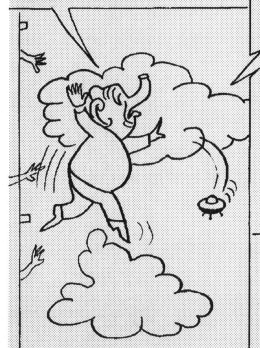

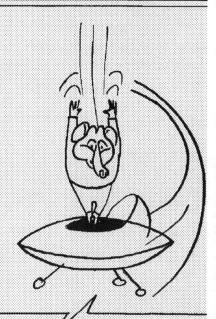

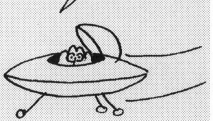

"Security is what this debate was all about. Everyone getting a health security card, which would guarantee all Americans access to a comprehensive package of benefits, no matter where they work, where they live, and whether or not they've ever been sick before."

The End

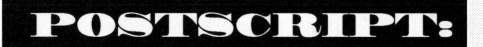

Where Are They Now?

HILLARY CLINTON went on to consider a career in politics;

DONALD DOLLERZ sold his lucrative practices and now travels worldwide with Mother Theresa, devoting himself full-time to what he describes as "the work of the soul";

GEORGE GOODHEART cut his hair and went back to school, recently receiving his M.B.A. from Wharton;

POINDEXTER PRUFROCK was last seen white water rafting in Southern Utah, singing the praises of the macrobiotic, stimulant- and mucus-free diet;

NOAH NOSTRUM does the Sumo wrestling circuit at various strip malls in the American midwest;

and **DORIS BROWN** remained herself.

INDEX

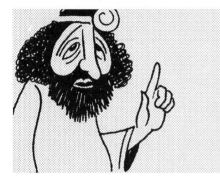
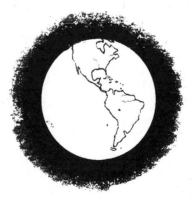

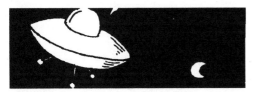

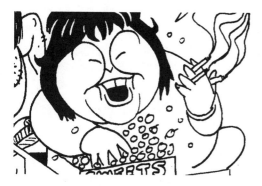

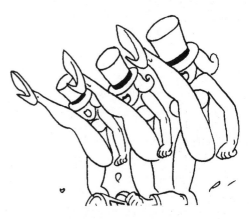

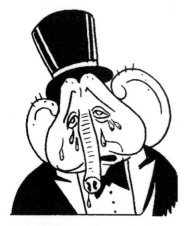

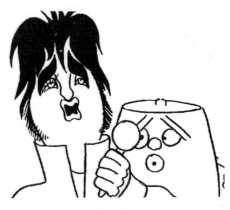